I. Chief of ₁

I CAME into the House one morning, great clad, for we subjects esteemed ourselves much on our great garments, and saw a man of honor talking whom I knew not, usually apparelled; for it was a plain material suit which appeared to have been made by an evil nation tailor; his cloth was plain and not extremely perfect, and I recollect a spot or two of blood upon his little band, which was very little bigger than a collar; his cap was without a hatband; his height was of a decent size; his sword adhered near his side; his face enlarged and ruddy; his voice sharp and untunable and his expressiveness loaded with fervour.

n these words the Royalist retainer, Sir Philip Warwick, recorded the impression which Oliver Cromwell made upon him that November morning. It was 1640; the spot Westminster. That mid year the King, Charles I, had driven a military to fight the Scots, and had been humiliatingly crushed — for the second time in a year. A détente left the Scots in charge of northern England. They were to be paid £850 every day until a last deal was finished up. In the event that the cash were not impending they would cross the Tees and walk south. Charles, poverty stricken, had to bring Parliament and submit to the Commons' requests for clearing change. It was to be a long parliament, the Long Parliament. Among the MPs was the part for Cambridge, Oliver Cromwell. As Sir Philip Warwick's noteworthy portrayal clarifies, in 1640 Cromwell was not a popular man; only a back-bencher whose garments were still nation made. However, this moderately aged country honorable man remained upon the edge of one of the most amazing political and military vocations in the entire of English history. Shocking and furthermore perplexing. How could it be that a man whose first experience of war came when he was 43 years old, who before this had gotten no tactical preparing, should end up being one of the world's extraordinary soldiers?

His political accomplishment was monstrous, obviously. Before the end he had, as his adversary Edward Hyde, Lord Clarendon, composed, 'mounted himself upon the lofty position of three realms, without the name of ruler yet with a more noteworthy power and authority than ever practiced or asserted by any ruler'. No big surprise Clarendon called him 'this uncommon man'. However his political achievement is less uncommon than his accomplishment in war. He was, all things considered, brought into the world to legislative issues, both in the nation and in Parliament. The Cromwells were one of the two families which overwhelmed the social and political life of

Huntingdonshire. No under eleven of the MPs in the Long Parliament were his cousins, including men as remarkable as John Hampden and Oliver St John. Despite the fact that in 1640 he was as yet unclear at the rich court of Charles I, he irrefutably had a place with the English decision class. Yet, he had not been destined to war; nor like numerous Englishmen, had he traveled to another country to battle. However he was to lead troops into fight against well known and experienced commandants — and beat them, once in a while, yet without fail. He was to construct a military and a naval force which made him, as the Duke of Tuscany put it, 'the fear of the entire world'. In the specialty of war he was unparalleled time permitting. Normally individuals considered what he may have done had he begun before throughout everyday life. Cromwell himself pondered as well. 'Is it accurate to say that i were pretty much as youthful as you,' he once commented to John Lambert, 'I ought not question, ere I passed on, to thump at the doors of Rome.'

Is it conceivable to clarify Cromwell's prosperity? Or on the other hand should we bow before the theoretical secret of individual virtuoso? Positively not many essayists have attempted to clarify it. There are many books on the Civil War; there are numerous books

— maybe too much — on Oliver Cromwell, the Puritan legislator. However not starting around 1899 when Lt Col T. S. Baldock distributed his Cromwell as a Soldier has there been a full-length study dedicated to this part of Cromwell's life. Very from the beginning there grew up a story that as a youngster he had battled for the Protestant reason in Germany. The story is altogether without establishment, yet by what other means could one clarify his later profession? Likely he read records of the techniques for fighting utilized so effectively by Gustavus Adolphus. Such records, distributed in The Swedish Intelligencer and The Swedish Soldier, were well known perusing in England during the 1630s. However, book perusing doesn't make soldiers. If we are to comprehend Cromwell the officer we should start by exploring three unique subjects. To start with, the idea of fighting in mid-seventeenth-century Europe. Second, the province of English society in 1640 — how much was England ready for war? Third, the personality of the man himself. Who was he, this chaotically dressed MP who kept 'his sword adhered near his side'?

Born on 25 April 1599, he had burned through the vast majority of the initial thirty years of his life in and around his origin, Huntingdon. It was a tranquil, even a dull market town set in the level wide open of the south east Midlands. Maybe the most astonishing thing to occur there was the yearly lesson against black magic, blessed by Oliver's granddad, Sir Henry Cromwell, whose spouse had been killed by a witch — or so Sir Henry believed.

In 1599 the Cromwell family was at the stature of its common achievement. Sir Henry Cromwell — prominently known as the Golden Knight — resided in sublime style in the extraordinary place of Hinchingbroke. It was here that his child, Sir Oliver Cromwell, sumptuously engaged King James on his advancement south from Edinburgh to climb the high position of England in 1603. As per later legend it was on the event of this visit that the four-year-old Oliver punched the nose of Prince Charles Stuart, later King Charles I, at the time only two years of age. We should not to trust this story, yet the topic of harshness and riotousness happens too often in the stories of Cromwell's adolescence and youth for it to be overlooked through and through. Unquestionably in later life he found in joking around some delivery from pressure. In 1648 a conversation about the eventual fate of the government finished in a pad battle. Also when that question was chosen, and Oliver Cromwell came to sign the warrant which sentenced the King horribly, he and one more of the appointed authorities were found inking each other's appearances with their pens, like the entire thing were only a student trick and, all things considered, somewhat simpler to bear. One pundit declared that Oliver's harshness was the consequence of his having been ruined by his mom, Elizabeth Steward of Ely. There is, obviously, no chance of telling, yet it's undeniably true that out of her seven enduring kids, just one, Oliver, was a kid. Oliver's dad, Robert Cromwell, was the second child of the Golden Knight and acquired from him a home worth some £300 per year. As a JP and as bailiff of the district of Huntingdon he was a man of some neighborhood significance, however particularly in the shadow of his lavish senior sibling out at Hinchingbroke. Thinking back Cromwell could say of himself that he was 'by birth a refined man residing neither in any impressive tallness nor yet in obscurity'.

He was taught, similar to Samuel Pepys, at the syntax school at Huntingdon, directly not too far off from the house where he resided. In Oliver's day the expert there was no customary schoolmaster. Thomas Beard, a Cambridge graduate and a Puritan priest, had, quite a while before he was delegated to Huntingdon, composed a popular book: The Theater of God's Judgements. The book considers life to be a battle among God and the powers of murkiness. The choose battle for God and, inasmuch as they comply with his laws, are sure of triumph. Verifiable occasions are deciphered as being (incidentally) awards for the authentic or (all the more frequently) as disciplines for the underhanded. These decisions are known as 'fortunes' — a word which repeats over and over in Cromwell's letters and talks. God's fortunes accept record of lords just as ordinary people. For sure in Beard's book great lords are uncommon animals. In all way of ways they could be viewed as needing and meriting rectification — assuming they burdened abusively, for instance, or on the other hand in the event that they assaulted private property. Cromwell certainly read this book, however regardless of whether it at any point became obvious youthful Oliver to view others' apples as sacrosanct private property is another matter. As indicated by one variant of his childhood his 'scrumping' was entirely famous, to the point that he procured the moniker of the Apple Dragon. Despite how this might be, there can be no question that Beard's philosophy was to be of far more prominent significance in Cromwell's later life than any Latin he figured out how to instruct him.

In 1616 Cromwell went to Cambridge. For a year he was an understudy in the Puritanical environment of Sidney Sussex College. Yet, Cromwell was never a researcher by disposition. What proof there is recommends that his favored subjects were math and history, however that in general he was 'more well known for his activities in the fields than in the schools, being one of the main intermediaries and players of football, bludgeons or some other riotous game or game'. He was said to have been 'effortlessly satisfied with study, taking more have a great time pony and field work out'. Probably it was in these years that he fostered his notable affection for hunting and selling. As a fruitful rangers officer his characteristics as a horseman need no stressing, and surprisingly a Royalist antiquarian commented upon the consideration which Cromwell took to see that his fighters were very much mounted and their ponies appropriately looked after.

He didn't remain long at Cambridge. In 1617 his dad passed on leaving Oliver at the top of a group of seven females. With obligations push right on time upon him it was concluded that he ought to go to London. As a landowner and in all likelihood a future JP he would should be comfortable with the precedent-based law. The spot to concentrate on this was one of the Inns of Court; for his situation it was most likely Lincoln's Inn, undeniably arranged in the fields between the City and the Palaces of Westminster and Whitehall. It offered him a chance of making associations and fellowships among the subjects, lawmakers, traders and agents who lived and dealt with one or the other side of Lincoln's Inn. So Cromwell joined the crowd of young fellows, the majority of them of a comparative age and station as himself, who were shaking to find the flight of stairs which would take them up in the world.

ne of the main strides on the flight of stairs of desire was a good
marriage. On 22 August 1620, only four months after his twenty-first birthday celebration, Oliver Cromwell wedded Elizabeth, oldest little girl of a rich City hide seller, Sir James Bourchier. The wedding occurred at St Giles' Church, Cripplegate, where somewhere in the range of fifty years after the fact the artist John Milton was to be covered. During the following eleven years Elizabeth bore seven kids, six of whom made due, four young men and two young ladies — a decent normal estimated family by seventeenth century guidelines. Elizabeth was to outlast her significant other, yet her ethics were private ones and she generally remained circumspectly behind the scenes. Noxious tattle recommended that Cromwell found different women more alluring — strikingly Frances Lambert, spouse of John Lambert who, during the 1650s, drafted a constitution called the Instrument of Government. As an embarrassment mongering life of Cromwell (distributed in 1663) put it: 'They say that the Lord Protector's Instrument is found under my Lady Lambert's underskirt'. Everything appears to be fairly unlikely. Following thirty years of marriage Oliver was as yet ready to keep in touch with Elizabeth: 'Really, in the event that I love you not very well, I think I blunder not then again much. Thou craftsmanship dearer to me than some other animal' however he proceeded to add, a little straight maybe, 'let that get the job done'. Indeed, even as the spouse of the Lord Protector she was to be a to some degree unremarkable figure, jokingly called Joan — the seventeenth-century name for a typical worker young lady. The one enduring letter composed by her does essentially nothing to adjust this impression. What is completely clear is that Cromwell settled on his own choices. He was not under his better half's thumb, as was claimed of a portion of his recognized counterparts, Sir Thomas Fairfax and Sir William Waller for instance. A mocking leaflet entitled Dreadful News in Hell (composed after the Restoration) reports a discourse between the apparition of Old Noll — Cromwell — his actually living spouse Joan. When she communicated a dread that she may be shipped off the Tower, her significant other's apparition simply said 'Why? You were never assistant to any of my horrible villainies, were ye?'

oon after the wedding Cromwell and his lady got back to Huntingdon. The years slipped discreetly by. Then, at that point, in 1630 the harmony was upset by 'dishonorable and improper addresses' made by Oliver Cromwell. The base of the difficulty lay in an endeavor by Huntingdon's decision club to fix their grip on the public authority of the town. Another illustrious contract was to liberate them from the need of looking for yearly re-appointment to office and to give them more noteworthy controls over the district's normal grounds. Driving the ones who exhibited against being accordingly denied of their freedoms as burgesses was Cromwell. The decision government went to the Crown for help. Cromwell was

pulled to Westminster and made to show up before the Lord Privy Seal. Looked by this blend of his nearby foes and the illustrious administration of Charles I, Cromwell had to give way. He needed to apologize, concede that his fights had been 'causeless and not well grounded' and his discourses made 'in hotness and energy'. Two years sooner, in 1628, Cromwell had been picked MP for Huntingdon, a man of developing impact in neighborhood issues. In any case, presently he was beaten. He could never sit for the ward again. In May 1631 he sold virtually the entirety of his Huntingdon property and moved to St Ives. Here as a sharecropper, as of now not a freeholder or a JP, he recovered. Crushed in his first fight, he considered emigrating to New England, yet ultimately chose to remain on in his dark backwater. The loss was even more unpleasant in light of the fact that in 1630 the Lord Privy Seal was Henry Montagu, Earl of Manchester, the one who had removed the Cromwells from their situation as the main family in the area. The most recent twenty years had been long periods of declining fortunes for the Cromwells; in 1627 Hinchingbroke itself had must be offered to the Montagus. Nobody might have imagined that under twenty years after the fact an individual from the cadet part of this declining family would be the most dreaded man in Europe.

The upswing in Cromwell's fortunes came in 1636. His mom's sibling, Sir Thomas Steward of Ely, made a will naming Oliver as his main beneficiary. Cromwell and his family moved to Ely, to a house arranged (as Thomas Carlyle put it) 'two discharges from the Cathedral'. Cromwell was currently a man of extensive riches — and a man more content with himself. For there is a decent arrangement of proof to recommend that lately he had been upset both as a main priority and body. As ahead of schedule as 1628 a specialist's casebook records that Cromwell was incredibly despairing, that his tissue was extremely dry and shriveled, that he had a constant aggravation in his left side and a stomach-throb for three hours after suppers. Different cures had been attempted, however without any result. Better outcomes were gotten on another event when Cromwell took a portion of mithridate to avert the plague and, causing him a deep sense of shock, observed that it got his face free from pimples. A subsequent specialist revealed that Cromwell used to call him out at the entire hours of the constantly in light of the fact that he accepted, altogether without legitimization, that he was kicking the bucket.

At different occasions he would lie indifferently in bed for a really long time. Glancing back at these years Cromwell himself wrote (in 1638 in a letter to his cousin): 'Favored be His Name for sparkling upon so dull a heart as mine! You know what my way of life hath been. Gracious I have lived in and cherished murkiness and despised the light. I was a chief,

the head of heathens. This is valid; I abhorred righteousness, yet God showed leniency toward me. O the wealth of His kindness!' As Christopher Hill has composed, 'regardless of whether there was any association between the wealth of uncle Thomas Steward and the wealth of God's leniency we will most likely never know'. In any occasion the two girls in what Cromwell called his 'second family' were brought into the world in 1637 and 1638. Cromwell's long periods of emergency were over.

Cromwell had gone through the Puritan strict experience known as change — a feeling of being in direct fellowship with God, a feeling of being 'saved'. From here on out Cromwell was certain that he was one of the 'holy people', one of God's choose, a man destined for paradise. There were times when his confidence provided him with a sensation of joy and power — this was his mind-set just before the Battle of Naseby. It provided him with a level of fearlessness which empowered him to move uninhibitedly in a universe of strict disarray and political vulnerability. Cromwell and his individual Puritans felt an inward impulse to act, to co-work in achieving God's motivations. Richard Hooker, a Church of England man who viewed these Puritans with grave doubt, called attention to that 'when the personalities of men are once wrongly convinced that it is the desire of God to have those things done which they extravagant, their viewpoints are as thistles in their sides, never enduring them to take rest till they have brought their hypotheses into training'. Hence in this world they were activists. At Doomsday, said John Bunyan, men will be asked not 'Did you accept?' however 'Were you practitioners, or talkers just?' 'Our rest we expect somewhere else,' composed Cromwell, and it lamented him that 'this being the reason for God and of his kin, such countless holy people ought to be in their security and ease, and not come out to crafted by the Lord in this extraordinary day of the Lord'.

Moreover men like Cromwell would in general feel that they were on the triumphant side — normally enough since they accepted they were taking care of God's responsibilities. In words taken from Tyndale's interpretation of the Bible, 'The Lord was with Joseph and he was a fortunate individual'. 'What weakling would not battle when he makes certain of triumph?' asked one Puritan. This was the stuff of which Cromwell's warriors were made.

For Puritans the main issue was to find exactly what God's motivations expected of them in some random circumstance. Somewhat this would be spread the word about for them thanks to occasions — 'provisions'. 'My dear companion, let us investigate fortunes' composed Cromwell when he was attempting to determine what ought to be the destiny of King Charles. However, how might they be investigated, and how deciphered? Normally it was enticing to see the way to

private benefit and portray it as the way delineated for you by God. 'Actually,' thought of one seventeenth-century diarist, 'I followed the call of fortune when it concurred with my humor and appeared to will generally respect and benefit; yet assuming that equivalent provision had called me to stop my better places and take me to meaner spots, or none by any stretch of the imagination, I had not really quickly and cheerily followed it.' Since Cromwell's fortune was continually calling him to better places it was very much simple for his foes to blame him for pietism. Clarendon, an adroit whenever biased spectator, composed: 'Cromwell, however the best dissembler living, consistently made his pietism of particular use and advantage to him'.

Be that as it may, regardless of whether you stayed away from pietism and personal responsibility, how is it that you could be certain which of a few potential approaches was the one expected by God? One potential reaction to this issue was: keep a watch out. In time the genuine importance of occasions would become more clear. It is this which clarifies Cromwell's ditherings at crucial points in time when he couldn't distinguish a huge example behind befuddled and clashing cross-flows of a complex political circumstance. In any case, when he saw what direction the tide was starting to stream then he moved — and moved determinedly and with an unmistakable heart. Hence in Cromwell's vocation we have this inquisitive mix of times of hesitation followed by rushed and regularly brutal activity. As in governmental issues so additionally in war. Cromwell depicted his own conduct at troublesome minutes in his missions as 'holding up upon the Lord, and not knowing what course to take, for without a doubt we know only what God pleaseth to show us of His incredible mercy'.

ut even in these times of uncertainty Cromwell didn't simply sit and pause. However for some time his blade might have dozed in his grasp, he didn't quit mental conflict. There was never a second's tranquility from the battle to get occasions and to perceive how God's motivation was dealing with them. This feeling of battle comes through unmistakably in a letter Cromwell directed to his secretary in 1645. As it was brought to him for his particular it talked about 'individuals of God all England over who have looked out for God for a gift'. Yet, this expression didn't exactly hit the imprint. Cromwell got his pen, crossed out the words 'looked out for' and modified it to peruse 'individuals of God all England over who have grappled with God for a gift'. This disposition submitted Cromwell to a critical examination of occasions and drove him to assess the hard realities of a circumstance prior to settling on a strategy. This by itself was sufficient to make him a definitely more practical legislator than King

Charles might ever be.

Puritan he without a doubt was, however it merits seeing that the viewpoint of a seventeenth-century Puritan was not really rigid in the advanced feeling of the word. During the 1640s numerous Puritan MPs couldn't be convinced to go to evening sittings since they liked to invest their energy at the theater, park or bowling green. Cromwell might have worked more diligently than a portion of the Puritans, however he likewise partook in his delights — regardless of whether a nation honorable man's hunting and selling, or the harsh commonsense jokes of a trooper among officers. His adoration for music drove him to set up an administration Committee for the Advancement of Music. He jumped at the chance to smoke and drink port (which he is said to have brought into England). His beloved brew cheered for the sake of 'Morning Dew'. If, as Lord Protector, he precluded race gatherings it was not on the grounds that he was against the game but since the horse racing was regularly a cover for rebellious meetings. In numerous ways our textbook generalization of the grouch Puritan is a bogus one — just a few Puritans were that way. Similarly bogus is the traditional image of Cromwell and his allies as Roundheads — men who wore dismal apparel and had their hair edited short. Cromwell and his companions were courteous fellows, and they wore their hair like noble men: shoulder length.

At Ely Cromwell indeed became engaged with nearby legislative issues and, as at Huntingdon, he took the side of his less fortunate neighbors. This time it was over the topic of depleting the Fens. Without a doubt it was important to expand the space of arable land to take care of the developing populace. However, the large organizations which did the work needed their benefit, so they saved an extent of the depleted land for themselves, while the helpless average people lost their privileges of pasturage, fishing and fowling. By 1637 Cromwell was related to the ordinary citizens' motivation. As per a grumbling against him, 'Mr Cromwell of Ely had attempted, the ordinary citizens paying him a groat for each cow they had upon the house, to hold the drainers in suit of law for quite a long time, and that meanwhile they ought to partake in each foot of their hall'. Simultaneously there were riots in the Fens. People, furnished with grass cutters and pitchforks, opposed the endeavors made to drive away their steers. By 1638 apprehensions of an overall resistance of the Fenlanders convinced the King to intercede. Charles reported that the everyday citizens could stay possessing their freedoms for the time being.

hree years after the fact, when Cromwell was a MP and more noteworthy issues were alarming the realm, Cromwell showed that he had not forgotten the

Fensmen. Some waste terrains close to St Ives had been encased and offered to the Earl of Manchester's child, Lord Mandeville. The ordinary people appealed to the House of Commons for review, however the Lords interceded for the Montagus. While the average people went rogue, recuperating ownership 'in a wild and warlike way', Cromwell talked about the undertaking in Parliament. He contended that the Lords' mediation was a break of Commons' advantages and he convinced the House to set up a board of trustees to think about the matter. The administrator of the board of trustees was Edward Hyde, and we have his threatening record of Cromwell's conduct as an individual from that council. Obviously he instructed the candidates and their observers in what they should say, 'then, at that point, backed and developed what they said with incredible energy'. Proof given on the opposite side was suffocated in the racket made by his men. At the point when Hyde attempted to quietness them, Cromwell blamed him for prejudice. In response to Lord Mandeville's assertion of his case Cromwell answered 'with such a lot of foulness and impoliteness, and in language so opposite and hostile … his entire carriage was so violent and his conduct so ill bred' that Hyde took steps to report him to the House.

Cromwell's determined and eager title of the reason for the Fenland ordinary people was to work well for him when the Civil War started. He approached the Fenlanders to wage war for 'the opportunity of the gospel and the rules that everyone must follow', however many individuals accepted that they followed Cromwell against the King 'the somewhat in light of the fact that they trust Parliament will give them their fens once more'. By 1643 the Royalists were calling him 'Master of the Fens'. They implied it jokingly, however the title is an update that by his remain on neighborhood issues Cromwell had gotten for himself a power base which was autonomous of the changes of political and dignified life at Westminster and Whitehall.

2. A Kind of Twilight

CROMWELL was never an expert fighter who passed on the legislative issues to different men. He didn't just do orders. In case he rode in the Valley of Death he knew the motivation behind why. He was battling for a purpose wherein he accepted, and not just in light of the fact that it was his responsibility to battle. In this Cromwell was not the slightest bit particular, for the English Civil War, as most respectful conflicts, was a conflict battled for specific standards of religion and government what men held to be significant. It was a conflict wherein government officials directed militaries and in which fighters thought that it is difficult to try not to become lawmakers regardless of whether they needed to. It was a conflict, not of endurance, but rather of causes. Maybe the best articulation of this fundamental reality about the conflict is the letter composed by Sir William Waller, a Parliamentarian, to his close buddy Sir Ralph Hopton, a Royalist. Under three weeks after the date of this letter the militaries directed by these two men conflicted in the savagely challenged Battle of Lansdown (July 1643).

To my Noble companion Sir Ralph Hopton at
Wells. Sr,
The experience I have had of your Worth, and the bliss I have appreciated in your kinship are woundinge contemplations when I view the current distance between us. Certainely my warm gestures to you are unchangeable to the point that aggression itselfe can't abuse my companionship in your individual, however I should be consistent with the reason wherein I serve; where my soul is intrigued, any remaining commitments are gobbled up. That incredible God, which is the searcher of my heart, knows with what miserable sence I goe upon this assistance, and with what an ideal disdain I despise this warr without an enemie. The God of harmony in his fun time send us harmony, and meanwhile fitt us to get it: Wee are both upon the stage and should act those parts that are alloted us in this Tragedy: Lett us do it in a method of honor, and without personall hostilities, at all the issue be, I will never eagerly surrender the dear title of
Your most affectionated
companion and faithfull
Servant
Wm. Waller
romwell was to end up in a comparative quandary. His very own portion

cousins became Royalists; and he waged war against them. Be that as it may, in 1640 nobody envisioned it would result in these present circumstances. Britain experienced been at harmony for so long

that men had lost the propensity for considering battle as a real part of the choices open to them. Accordingly they floated into it without seeing where they were going. At the kickoff of the Long Parliament men who might thereafter battle on inverse sides were joined in their assurance to change the Government and render unimaginable those practices which had been so difficult during the Eleven Years' Tyranny — the eleven years (1629-40) when Charles I managed without a parliament. The disliked privilege courts were abrogated. Parliamentary command over customs contribution was re-attested and all tax collection without assent was announced illicit. One rule broadcasted that this parliament couldn't be broken up besides with its own assent, while one more guaranteed that there would be continuous meetings later on. Cromwell's part in this work was that of the 'great council man' — he sat on no under eighteen. However in no way, shape or form in the front position of the Commons chiefs, not a Pym or a Hampden, unmistakably he was a significant man. At the point when Sir Philip Warwick watched him talking, he saw that 'he was particularly noticed unto'. Given his experience and family associations it was normal that Cromwell ought to be a skillful Parliamentarian.

At this stage he was primarily worried about strict issues. He had a place with the extreme Puritan minority which, in the late spring of 1641, squeezed for the abrogation of diocesans, or possibly for their rejection from the House of Lords. On such inquiries, the once joined Commons was miserably isolated. For some time just the presence of the Scottish armed force kept Charles from tracking down a method for liberating himself from this problematic Parliament. Then, at that point, in September 1641 the hotly anticipated arrangement with the Scots was finished up. The Scottish armed force pulled out across the Tweed and left the Commons unprotected. The drive lay with the King. Moderate assessment had swung back to his side and there was a broadly felt trust that he could make a new beginning based on the great laws to which he had given his assent.

Then, with insane speed, came news which changed the whole circumstance. The Catholic locals of Ulster rose up against the English and Scottish pioneers who had taken their properties. The development spread like quickly and soon the entire of Protestant Ireland was nearly being lost. In England the fall of 1641 was loaded up with bits of hearsay and barbarity stories. Huge number of men, ladies and youngsters were said to have been killed

— simmered alive or conveyed to the ocean in flawed boats. Others were stripped and passed on to pass on of openness. The legend of the Irish slaughters was born.indeed this insubordination was most likely no nastier than some other defiance — the

revolts unquestionably had cause enough to wage war, yet this isn't the manner in which it looked to Englishmen during the 1640s. They accepted that the Irish were scarcely human. All were concurred that the socially mediocre Irish should be decreased to their legitimate condition of subjection to the English. A military must be raised
— yet who might control it, King or Commons? Could Charles be entrusted with a military? For what reason did the Ulster rebels display a commission from the King, approving them to hold onto the grounds of the Protestant pilgrims? The archive was a fraud, however it is huge that there were individuals who accepted that Charles was able to do something like this. When he had a military may he not use it to overawe Parliament and fix all the great work of the last year? Could the King be trusted? This was the main point of contention over what men isolated, and over which common conflict broke out.Religious contrasts, albeit significant and especially troubling during a time which felt the requirement for solidarity and consistency, would not have caused a conflict. In a perfect world the nation was represented by King and upper class joined in political marriage. However, John Pym's gathering was worried about the possibility that that assuming the King were given command over a military then he would sort out a shotgun separate and henceforward rule alone. They were not ready to see a re-visitation of the Eleven Years' Tyranny.

There is no question where Cromwell remained on the topic of the military. On 6 November 1641 he presented a movement to give the Puritan Earl of Essex ability to order every one of the trainbands south of the Trent. The accompanying fortnight was taken up by the wild discussion over the Grand Remonstrance — a long and itemized prosecution of fifteen years of mismanagement under Charles I. After a turbulent meeting finishing at the then exceptional hour of two AM of 23 November the Remonstrance was in the end conveyed by 159 votes to 148. An onlooker of the conflicts which happened in the House that evening composed: 'I thought we had all sat in the valley of the shadow of death'. Furthermore coming back Cromwell was heard to say that assuming the Remonstrance had been dismissed he would have sold all he had and gone to America.

After the Grand Remonstrance had been printed and flowed there could be no hiding the profound divisions inside the country. Over the Christmas occasion the crowd, driven by London disciples, attacked Westminster, revolting and yelling 'No priests', 'No Popish Lords'. The understudies were derisively excused as 'Roundheads' — for among the guidelines overseeing a disciple's life were rules against marriage, sex and long hair.

In answer the King's officers watching Westminster were called Caballeros — which means Spanish troopers, men who killed Protestants. Just later did the word 'Careless' come to infer valor rather than ruthlessness. A handout author in 1642 provides us with some thought of what 'Carefree' implied around then. It alludes to 'that Legion of Devils, that pile of rubbish and drosse and trash of the land, comprised of Jesuits, and Papists and Atheists, that grisly and butcherly Generation regularly knowne by the name of Cavaliers'. In this air of dread and vulnerability gossipy tidbits about plot and counter-plot duplicated. However, there was still no thoughtful conflict. Albeit the two sides dreaded the aims of the other, neither had at this point straightforwardly engaged force.

All this changed on the evening of 4 January 1642. At the top of a few hundred horsemen Charles rode to the House of Commons to capture five individuals — Pym, Hampden, Haselrig, Holles and Strode — on charges of conspiracy. In spite of the fact that he left his continuing in the hall of the House, and removed his cap as he entered, the entryways were left open so the individuals could see the outfitted officers. However, Pym had been admonished and had, by and by, out-moved the King. The five individuals got away from in the nick of time. 'Every one of my birds have flown.' Charles' despondent words were an affirmation that his overthrow had fizzled, and that he no longer realized what to do. On 10 January the King left his capital. He would not see it again except if he came as a successful general or as a detainee in the possession of his foes. Just presently was unmistakably the issue would be settled by an enticement for arms.

Like John Pym, Cromwell rushed to draw the example of these occasions. On 14 January he moved that a board of trustees ought to be set up to think about the safeguard of the realm. He had a functioning influence occupied with fund-raising and troops — apparently for the concealment of the Irish resistance, yet maybe likewise with an eye to the weakening circumstance at home. Cromwell himself bought in £2000 to an organization which should back a military for Ireland and afterward repay itself out of agitators' seized domains. Along these lines concealment of revolt and a beneficial piece of property theory were to go inseparably — obviously. In any case, Irish issues would need to stand by; there was seriously squeezing business to hand. Charles wouldn't give his consent to a Militia Bill which gave Parliament command over the nation's military, so in March 1642 the two Houses gave it as a statute, guaranteeing for it the full powers of law. Here, finally, was the progressive demonstration, the grip at parliamentary administrative power. In spite of the fact that couriers nominations actually kept on passing between arrangements were pointed not such a huge amount at compromise as at causing the opposite side to seem answerable for the breakdown. They discussed harmony and ready for war.

For both the main fundamental was to hold onto control of the magazines in which arms and ammo were put away. Now and again the competition to control the magazines formed into furnished conflicts — at Leicester, at Manchester and at Hull. Structure was not simply a magazine. In the event that Charles held it he had a port of section for the unfamiliar armed force which the Queen, presently at the Hague, was striving to gather. However, on two events in the spring and summer of 1642 Hull blamed him for out. As these nearby battles erupted all around the nation Cromwell's musings went normally to his own constituents at Cambridge.

Like the nation all in all, Cambridge itself was parted into two groups; here without a doubt the political divisions were elevated by customary college transplants and locals competition. The residents would in general help Parliament while the schools stayed faithful to the King. In July Cromwell sent £100 worth of arms at his own cost to the metropolitan volunteers — and they observed that terminating through school windows made arms drill considerably more agreeable. The scholastics in the interim had weapons raised from London and put away in the schools' vaults. They additionally gathered cash and sent it on to the King. Energized by these indications of their steadfastness Charles kept in touch with the bad habit chancellor of the college and welcomed the universities to give up their silver plate to him 'for safety's sake'. Chief James Dowcra was sent with an organization of officers to accompany this significant freight to York. Cromwell, notwithstanding, was cautioned of the risk. Toward the beginning of August he hustled along from London, brought a power up in western Cambridgeshire, captured a portion of the plate out and about and held onto Cambridge Castle. Dowcra was captured and had his ponies seized. By possessing the palace, Cromwell not just acquired a significant magazine, he likewise shut the street out from Cambridge thus forestalled further endeavors to move the plate. On 15 August the Committee of Defense declared to the House of Commons that 'Mr Cromwell has held onto the Magazine in the Castle at Cambridge and hath prevented the diverting of the plate from that University; which, as some report, was to the worth of £20,000 or thereabouts'.

But this activity, quick and viable idea it was, had in no way, shape or form settled the battle for control of Cambridge. While Cromwell held the palace, the Royalist sheriff, Sir John Cotton, gathered the district prepared band at King's College. Is it safe to say that they were at war or not? To one pamphleteer it appeared to be that 'we

lived in a sort of sundown … an overcast and hazy clime of pity and vulnerability'. Then, at that point, on 22 August 1642, the obscurity of vulnerability lifted. Ruler Charles increased his expectation at Nottingham and in this way lawfully made a condition of war. He sent the Earl of Carlisle and Sir John Russell to Cambridge with a commission to raise troops for his benefit. Cromwell saw that he wanted external assistance if he somehow happened to keep the shire from slipping into Royalist hands. At his solicitation 500 London dragoons were requested to Cambridge. They showed up on 30 August. These fortifications demonstrated definitive. Regardless of some backwater opposition in the universities and in the Isle of Ely, the shire remained solidly in Parliament's grip from this point forward. The assets of the City of London had influenced the situation in an equitably ready challenge between nearby powers. As MP, the connection man among Cambridge and London, Cromwell had played an imperative part.

s consistently couple of individuals needed conflict. From Yorkshire down to Devon and Cornwall there was an entire series of endeavors to make nearby arrangements of lack of bias and non-support. All fizzled. Hardly any individuals needed conflict, however less still confided in the opposite side adequately for harmony to be conceivable. Would-be neutrals were questioned by the two sides and to save their bequests from seizure they needed to pronounce their devotion for sure. There were numerous hesitant warriors — like the unwarlike Earl of Dorset, to whom the accompanying lines were attributed:

I can't act an officer's part
Nor freezing lie in trenches
But wish myself with everything
that is in me At Chelsey with my
wenches.

ven the people who figured out how to stay away from direct interest in the real business of battling became associated with the tensions of war some way or another, regardless of whether it was through billetting troops, work on fortresses or paying the incomprehensibly expanded tax collection made essential by war. Of the ones who battled some just followed their rulers, or picked the side which they thought would win. Yet, many followed their inner voice and decided in the light of the political and strict battles of the most recent two years. As indicated by his better half, Colonel Hutchinson read the declarations of the two players until 'he turned out to be richly educated in his arrangement and persuaded in his heart of the uprightness of the Parliament's motivation in place of common right'. 'What incredible matter is it to color for your God, a little before your time,' cried one East Anglian Puritan serve, 'Who might reside when Religion is dead?' In a

enrolling discourse he made in the commercial center at Huntingdon, Cromwell let his crowd know that he was battling 'for the freedom of the Gospel and the laws of the land'.

So, for some explanation, the nation favored one side. The decision class was divided directly into equal parts. Most companions upheld the King while, then again, most of vendors favored Parliament. The landed nobility were decently uniformly isolated. Topographically Parliament ordinarily controlled the region south and east of an unpredictable line attracted from the Humber to the Severn. It is broadly accepted that Parliament instructed the more extravagant portion of England and that, accordingly, its triumph was inescapable. In any case, this is to think little of the monetary assets of the Royalist respectability; the significance of the modern spaces of the west Midlands, South Wales and the Forest of Dean; and the worth of the provisions of arms which the King acquired from abroad and which were transported in through Newcastle, Bristol and the ports of the south west. This implied that the Royalists couldn't fault their losses in 1645 on a deficiency of war material. They were also prepared similar to the Parliamentary armed forces. The facts may show that Parliament directed the more noteworthy expected assets and that, over the long haul, these stores of solidarity would demonstrate definitive. However, the truth of the matter is that there was no since quite a while ago run. Inside three years the conflict was, to all aims and purposes, wrapped up. Parliament won, however it was not monetary geology which had determined the end result. What made a difference were the activities and abilities of men — in governmental issues, organization and, eventually, in war.

3. The Disciplines of War

THE English guest to the mainland can barely neglect to be struck by a repetitive element of European urban areas which is independently missing from those of his own country. Over and over the downtown area — the site of the old middle age town — is isolated from present day modern and private rural areas by a ring of wide avenues or by a wonderful support of yards and nurseries, a sort of smaller than expected green belt. In any case, English towns don't adjust to this normal European example. Here, as yet looking straight at us, we have one of the keys to understanding Cromwell's momentous profession as an officer. This 'green belt' is the site of previous city guards, not the archaic dividers, but rather the progressive fortresses which were included early current occasions. High stone dividers which had functioned admirably in the age of the ballista and crossbow were really defenseless against the new danger presented by weapons. It is sufficiently simple to be scorching around sixteenth-and seventeenth-century mounted guns. Garrett Mattingley, for instance, composed that 'the most experienced heavy weapons specialist may wonder whether or not to foresee whether when next he discharged it his firearm would send its fired straightforwardly to the objective, drop it with a kind of debilitate burp two or three hundred feet ahead, or explode the break, presumably killing him and his group'. Regardless as right on time as the finish of the fifteenth century weapons were truth be told equipped for conveying a sensibly exact level blow from long reach. The reaction of military designers and architects was to foster the stronghold, a squat fortress made from rubble and block which retained cannon shot, rather than cracking on sway as stone did. By opposing the new mounted guns and giving a stage to its very own weighty weapon, the stronghold definitely changed the current example of warfare.

An all around sustained and rich city could hope to have however many firearms as a military; for sure by an arrangement of commonly supporting outworks, with names like half-moons and horn-works, the city could contact challenge any besieger. This framework ended up being entirely successful, to the point that it was taken on by many states throughout the sixteenth century. Subsequently the European town, from the Baltic toward the North African coast, took on another appearance. To be sure any place Europeans settled abroad, from the Caribbean to India, they assembled towns which adjusted to this essential example; at Havana, Mombasa, Goa. As has been properly said, the stronghold was 'the most huge of all engineering structures advanced during the Renaissance'. In any case, except for a couple of spots like Carlisle and Berwick-on-Tweed in the fierce Border

country, English towns stayed resistant to the interests of this worldwide style. Laurence Sterne's Uncle Toby fell captivated. A large number of pages of Tristram Shandy is given to his excitement for half-moons, ravelins and crown-works, yet he was always unable to see the genuine article in England. All things being equal, on the bowling green, he needed to assemble his models of mainland towns.

England in Cromwell's time was a curiously unfortified nation and its uniqueness in this regard requires clarification. The ocean, obviously, kept unfamiliar trespassers under control and since the time the twelfth century the brought together managerial framework had empowered the lords to maintain order all through their little domain. Just in Wales and in Scotland did the visionaries keep on flourishing. In this manner on those events — uncommon by mainland standards

— when common conflict broke out, the conflicts which came about, the Wars of the Roses for instance, were battles of fights, not of attacks. The Tudors worked hectically to keep things much as they had consistently been; prosperous and dull, a general public untroubled by the possibility of war. So it stayed until January 1642. As one MP composed, 'It is peculiar to take note of how we have torpidly slid into this start of a common conflict, by one sudden mishap after another, as influxes of the ocean, which have presented to us this far; and we scant ability, however from paper battles we are currently gone to the subject of raising powers and naming a General and officials of a military'. By then it was past the point of no return. Town specialists quickly hurled what strongholds they could, yet in a few furious years they couldn't complete crafted by a century, particularly since the requests of armed force administration and war tax collection left them shy of the two men and cash. Accordingly once the different sides had outfitted themselves with sufficient attack big guns, however this set aside time obviously, there were not many towns — Oxford, the King's base camp, was one — which were fit to stand a genuine attack. At Winchester in 1645, for instance, the battering firearms required just a day to make a break in the dividers wide enough for thirty men abreast. What this implied was that a conflict battled in England could be something altogether different from battle on the landmass. Abroad a triumph over foe powers in the field did barely anything to tackle the issue of his strengthened towns. These typically must be famished into accommodation. However, barricades took such a long time that the crushed side had a lot of time to recuperate its solidarity and summon another military. Fights were thusly fairly trivial; to be sure numerous contemporary scholars censured them if all else fails of the clumsy or unfortunate

administrator. What fights there were typically occurred when a military went to the help of a barred town. In the English Civil War this is valid just of the Battle of Marston Moor. On the mainland war was predominantly a question of arduous barricades in which there was barely anything for the mounted force to do. It was the infantry which made a difference; even aristocrats battled as troopers. Thus wars continued for quite a while; for instance, the Thirty Years War (1618-48) in Germany, the eighty years' conflict among Spain and the Netherlands. For all his strategic advancements, intended to work on the portability of his soldiers, and for all his excitement to give fight, not even the incomparable Swedish general, King Gustavus Adolphus, could break out of the imperatives of this kind of fighting. At Nürnberg, in the late spring of 1632 for instance, he and Wallenstein invigorated their camps and afterward essentially stayed there, skirmishing around the stockpile lines to see whose arrangements gave out first.

y contrast the English circumstance was very unique. As Defoe wrote in his *emoirs of a Cavalier:*

I accept I might provoke every one of the Historians in Europe to tell me of any conflict in the World where, over the course of about four years, there were such countless pitched Battles, Sieges, Fights and Skirmishes, as in this War; we never digs in or settled in, never invigorated the Avenues to our posts ... 'Twas the overall Maxim of this War, Where is the Enemy? Release us and battle them ... I can't say 'twas the Prudence of the Parties, and had the King battled less he had acquired ... This Benefit anyway occurred overall to the Country, that it made a fast, however a ridiculous End, of the War, which in any case had kept going till it may have destroyed the entire Nation.

n England, indeed, the conflict was chosen by two fights inside the space of five weeks in the late spring of 1645 — to the consternation, maybe, of a portion of those expert troopers who had come to England looking for business and who accepted that, all around made due, the conflict may most recent twenty years. Furthermore in these two fights, Naseby and Langport, the definitive arm was the cavalry.

In the light of this difference it isn't sufficient to say, as Brigadier Peter Young, one of the most notable of present day antiquarians of the Civil War, has said, that 'fair officers love to secure men up fortifications ... the surest way to triumph is to start by annihilating the adversary's fundamental powers in the field. That done, even the most grounded strongholds will undoubtedly fall over the long haul.' This is to compose of seventeenth century fighting like it were post-Napoleonic, post-Industrial Revolution fighting. It happens additionally to be valid of

seventeenth-century England, however it isn't valid for a large portion of the seventeenth-century fighting, which was battled on the mainland. This also had its impact on the Civil War since definitely English administrators started by seeking Europe for their illustrations in the specialty of war. They needed to look some place — for as Defoe composed, in1697, while pushing the foundation of a tactical institute in England, 'men are not brought into the world with guns on their shoulders, nor fortresses in their minds' — and what other place could they look?

Although to a contemporary onlooker it appeared to be that their absence of military experience had 'effeminated' the English, this proved unable, truth be told, be said to describe all Englishmen. The people who delighted in soldiering, similar to the anecdotal saint of Defoe's Memoirs of a Cavalier, traveled to another country to battle: to France, Italy, Germany and, most importantly, to the Netherlands. In 1635 there were almost 10,000 men in the four English regiments utilized by the Dutch Republic. Normally a large portion of the leaders on the two sides of the Civil War were men with experience of battle on the mainland: the Fairfaxes, Essex, Waller, Prince Rupert, Goring, Hopton. The most clear special cases for this standard were extraordinary aristocrats like Manchester and Newcastle. Just Oliver Cromwell was to owe his position neither to high position nor to past experience. Oddly it is conceivable that his absence of involvement was really a benefit. In the seventeenth century war was turning into an undeniably proficient and logical business. The specialized intricacy of guns and the complexity of some combat zone moves implied that warriors must be very much bored. Their officials needed to prepare them just as lead them. Great officials consequently expected to dominate numerous abilities. To help them John of Nassau established, in 1616, the principal military institute in European history. For the people who couldn't go to a school of battle there was a developing number of books. In one such manual it took two pages to clarify exactly what was implied by the request 'right turn', which isn't is really to be expected considering the way that it here and there implied turn left! An official who had retained this information and whose learning was supported by experience in a battlefield where the study of fortresses and bars ruled, may have thought that it is hard to change his brain to new conditions. Assuming warriors are still some of the time leaned to battle the current conflict with the techniques for the final remaining one, it was just normal that they ought to have endeavored to take up arms in England as indicated by the very much attempted strategies for the landmass. Subsequently when Charles' nephew, the 23 year-old Prince Rupert, shown up in England in 1642, straight from his involvement with Germany and solid on the hypothesis of battle as a

consequence of the perusing he did during three years' detainment, he encouraged the King to invigorate his towns and develop the fortitude of his infantry. Rupert's vocation is an exceptionally enlightening one. He came to

England as a recognized master in the unobtrusive specialty of attack fighting. He left it with the standing of a swank rangers administrator. In England, the incredible officers, men like Rupert and Cromwell, were to become well known for the manner in which they dealt with cavalry in the fieriness of fight. Yet, when these two met, it was Cromwell who ended up being the master.

In England, then, at that point, restricting militaries searched each other out 'with such energy', in Defoe's expression, 'as though they had been in scramble to have their Brains knock'd out'. The conflict relied on the result of pitched fights. Subsequently two matters were indispensably significant. Initially the capacity of the soldiers to perform well in fight conditions. Besides the ability of the administrators who needed to choose when and where to submit their warriors to the frantically chancy business of battle.

On the first of these issues unmistakably, toward the start of the conflict, the soldiers were poor. There were not many prepared officers in England. The volunteer army arrangement of home guard implied that every province was to give the public authority 'prepared groups' — spare-time fighters who did a little light drill on Sunday mornings after chapel. Anyway well, or severely, the framework might have worked in Elizabeth's rule, by the 1630s it had obviously separated. As indicated by grumblings voiced by Colonel Ward in 1639 the one thing the prepared groups were truly prepared to do was to drink. The God they loved in their preparation, as another essayist put it, was not Mars yet Bacchus. The feelings of dread of these pundits were demonstrated very well indeed established by the presentation of King Charles' armed forces in the Scottish conflicts. 'I daresay,' composed Sir Edmund Verney, 'there was never so crude, so unskilful, thus reluctant an army.'

t was very little better during the 1640s. Sir William Waller found the prepared groups of Essex and Hertfordshire miserably mutinous. 'Such men,' he composed, 'are just fit for a scaffold here and a damnation from this point forward.' The one exemption for the standard of the alcoholic and jumbled prepared groups were those outfitted by London. They did their drill in the Artillery Garden at Bishopsgate or the Military Garden in St Martin's Fields. Obviously, they were taunted at for their agonies. In Beaumont and Fletcher's play The Knight of the Burning Pestle, a London prepared band skipper delivers a discourse to his officers. 'Men of their word, compatriots, companions, and my kindred officers. I have brought you this day from the shops of safety and the counters of content, to allot honor by the ell and ability by the pound.'

But the Londoners treated their soldiering in a serious way — and they murmured the play off the stage. It was also for Parliament that they accomplished for the conflict had barely begun when they alone remained between King Charles and the fast triumph he had anticipated. However not even the Londoners could fill in as the core of an ordinary armed force. They would guard their city, even walk similar to Gloucester; yet half a month from home was however much they could make due. During the missions of 1643 and 1644 Sir William Waller became progressively exasperated by what he called their old melody of 'Home! Home!' and on something like one event had to threaten to 'gun any of them that should utilize that base language'. One hateful eyewitness accepted that they were all the way out of their profundity once they abandoned the city. 'You ought to have seen the Londoners hurried to see what way of things cows were,' he composed. 'Some of them would say they had every one of them horns and would do incredible underhandedness.' But it was the tensions of family life rather than the dread of the field which caused problems for the Londoners. It is sufficiently simple to envision the sensations of a blustery officer, following a stormy night's rest in an open field, gotten a letter like the following:

Most deare and adoring husbane, my King love, — I recollect unto you, trusting that you are healthy as I ame at the writting heareof. My little Willie have bene wiped out this forknight. I implore you to come whome, in the event that youe stick cum saffly. I doo marfull that I can't heare from you ass well other naybores do. I implore youe to send me word when youe doo thinke youe shalt returne. You doe not consider I ame a solitary woemane; I figured you could never leave me thuse long togeder, so I rest evere petitioning God for your savese returne. Your caring spouse, Susan Rodway. Steadily petitioning God for you till deth I depart.

Yet whatever their concerns and deficiencies, in 1642 the prepared groups were the closest thing there was to a standing armed force. This clarifies the significance of the Militia Bill in the squabble among Charles and the Commons.

In the beginning phases of the conflict the two militaries depended vigorously on organizations and regiments raised by individual aristocrats and respectable men from their own tenantry and neighborhood. Numerous Royalist commandants paid their regiments out of their own pockets. The Earl of Worcester might have spent as much as £900,000; the Duke of Newcastle £800,000. Such men did not

resent the cash they spilled out for the King's sake. 'Had I a huge number of crowns and scores of children,' composed Lord Goring to his better half, 'the

King and his motivation ought to have them all.' Cromwell was luckier. He was one of the eighty Parliamentary chiefs who each got an award of £1,104 for raising a group of sixty pony. Then again he had likewise contributed an incredible arrangement to the asset out of which these awards were paid. He was supported recorded as a hard copy, as he did to Oliver St John in 1643: 'I have minimal expenditure of my own to help my troopers. My home is nearly nothing. I tell you, the matter of Ireland and England hath had of me, in cash, somewhere in the range of eleven and twelve hundred pounds. You have had my cash: I trust in God I want to wander my skin.' This aggregate was presumably comparable to Cromwell's pay more than a long term period.

One inconvenience of this primitive procedure for raising soldiers was that many skippers normally came to view their units as their own property. They were hesitant to fill holes in the positions by getting 'untouchables; subsequently many organizations were well underneath strength. What's more they detested proficient warriors, frequently their social inferiors, instructing them with their own men. They needed discipline. Sir Ralph Hopton whined that the gather of the Royalist powers in Devon was 'somewhat like an incredible reasonable ... every one of the Gentlemen of the County being so shipped with the cheer of the thing'.

One outward indication of this proprietorial disposition was the way that regiments were wearing whatever way and shading satisfied their colonel. John Hampden's men wore green coats, Lord Brooke's donned purple, Lord Saye's blue, etc. The main general request requiring a uniform tone for the entire armed force came in 1645 with the arrangement of the New Model Army. It was the main such request in European history, and from that date straight up to the First World War British soldiers wore red coats. Some contemporary assessment was against the uniform in light of the fact that assuming the individual were permitted to pick his own delicacy, crest and splendid tones he was bound to battle with soul and goal. Yet, such opportunity of fashion articulation made problems.

without even a trace of appropriate regalia, fights could undoubtedly become befuddled, with men not exactly certain who was battling on which side. So preceding a fight the armed forces embraced 'field signs'. The Parliamentarians, for instance, wore orange scarves at Edgehill, some green foliage in their caps at Newbury, and white cloths at Marston Moor. Moreover the 'field word' was additionally given out, on the off chance that anybody lost his cap or in the event that it was

important to challenge a man associated with wearing a bogus field sign. At

Naseby the King's statement was 'Sovereign Mary' and Fairfax's was 'God our Strength'. At Dunbar Cromwell's statement was 'The Lord of Hosts'. Part of the tangle at the Battle of Cheriton (March 1644) was brought about by the two sides wearing white tokens and embracing a similar field word: 'God with us'. The renowned song singing of the Parliamentary warriors could likewise assist with recognizing companion from adversary, as we can see from an occurrence during the Battle of Marston Moor depicted by a contemporary writer. The Royalists were routed:

... and in their flying and dissipating about, a large number of them ran most frightedly and amazedly to where a portion of the regiments of pony of the Parliament side were remaining wary, and all or the vast majority of their riders were strictly singing of Psalms, to whom the aforementioned wanderers of the adversary drew close and by their singing of Psalms seeing what their identity was, they all most furiously escaped back once more, and shouted out, 'God damn them, they had prefer to have been taken by the Parliament Roundheads.' For they just knew them, I say, to be the Parliament officers by their singing of Psalms. A favored identification and discernment indeed.

Perhaps the most smart of all field signs was that given by General Monck at the attack of Dundee in 1651. His fighters needed to have 'a white material or shirt hanging out behind'. This guaranteed that they had the most grounded conceivable intention in holding their countenances to the adversary; assuming they retreated in fear they could be confused with the foe. The militaries contained both cavalry and infantrymen, normally 33% or one-quarter mounted force to 66% or 3/4 infantry, however on the Royalist side by 1644 the extent of rangers was typically higher than this. The infantry comprised of pikemen (33%) and musketeers (66%). The musketeers' weapon was a gag stacking matchlock black powder gun shooting a weighty slug — twelve to the pound was the standard weight. Despite the fact that it had a scope of 400 yards or more, for genuine precision fire must be kept until the adversary was just 100 yards away. The musketeer conveyed his projectiles in a little pocket, yet in fight generally kept a couple in his mouth for accommodation in stacking. He additionally conveyed twelve charges of powder instant up in tube-molded cases made of tin or wood which dangled from a cowhide belt worn over the shoulder. This was known as a bandolier. Sadly in blustery climate or on the walk the bandoliers shook so noisily that it was beyond difficult to overwhelm the foe. During the Hispaniola undertaking of 1655 the warriors seldom had an unbroken night's rest. On numerous occasions their guards gave the alert, accepting that they could hear the shaking bandoliers of the propelling Spanish. After looking into it further the 'Spaniards' ended up being landcrabs, clicking their legs together.

In request to fire the gun a length of match was required. This was rope made of turned strands of tow and bubbled in vinegar or absorbed saltpeter. Each musketeer conveyed a loop of a few yards of it, held tight his belt, and a more limited piece, a few feet in length, in his left hand. At whatever point the adversary was close to he kept this piece lit at the two closures, prepared for quick firing

— difficult in wet climate. By requesting a sunrise assault at Dunbar in 1650 Cromwell fell upon the Scots before a significant number of their musketeers had struck their matches. Then again on the off chance that they had kept them land for the duration of the night they would quickly have run out of rope. Sir Ralph Hopton ended up in this dilemma on one event. He was being blockaded in Devizes by his companion Waller. He made do by sending his officials 'to look through each house in the town and to take all the bed-strings they could find, and to make them be rapidly beaten and bubbled'. The lit matches were, obviously, perilous. A flash from a match could burn down one of the charges in a man's bandolier, detonate them all, and kill the wearer. However, they could likewise be valuable. A skipper who wished to do a night retreat could leave lit matches behind in the desire for fooling his adversary into accepting that he was still there. By a similar token, regardless of whether the bandoliers clatter, lit matches made it difficult for musketeers to dispatch an unexpected night-assault. Normally the rest kept officers from the Hispaniola campaign had horrendous difficulty in differentiating between Spanish musketeers and discharge flies.

hat with the actual firearm, the match, the powder charges, the shots and in some cases a rest too, the musketeer had his hands full. To load, fire and yet again load all set aside time just as a decent arrangement of smoothness; a few adjusts a moment, best case scenario. Hence musketeers had typically been drawn up five, six or even ten profound. The front position terminated, then, at that point, walked back to the back and reloaded while the other at least four positions went through a similar move. However, Gustavus Adolphus found that gun discharge was undeniably more viable in case the musketeers generally shot together. So he prepared his men to frame three positions, the main position stooping, the second inclining forward, the third standing upstanding and pointing over the shoulders of the second. As such they terminated 'salvos' rather than the random moving fire created by the countermarch frameworks. Prior to taking part in fight the leaders attempted 'to get the breeze' of the foe. This was a development intended to get into a position where the breeze blew the smoke of the adversary's weapons and rifle once again into the eyes of his own troops.

It was generally extremely convoluted, however on the off chance that did effectively the musketeer could convey a deadly rocket: the protective layer penetrating projectile. In addition, albeit seventeenth-century specialists had the option to adapt to the injuries caused by a sword or a pike, they were defenseless assuming the bone was broken, or on the other hand if interior draining or blood-harming happened — conditions usually connected with shot injuries. On the off chance that a man wore covering, splinters of metal, just as the actual shot, may be crashed into his tissue. This happened to Sir Philip Skippon, one of the Parliamentary administrators, at the Battle of Naseby. As time passed by men acknowledged increasingly more unmistakably that there was little point in wearing substantial shield; in any case it was so costly. Different men contended that since not many black powder rifle balls really hit their objective it was an exercise in futility stressing over them. One reason for the infamous mistake of their shoot was clarified by Lord Orrery who saw English musketeers in real life in Ireland:

hose troopers which remove shots from their mouths (which is the nimblest way) or out of their pockets (which is slow) only here and there put any paper, tow or grass to slam the slug in; by which on the off chance that they discharge above bosom high the projectile disregards the top of the foe, and assuming they point low, the shot exits ere the flintlock is shot; and 'tis to this that I property the little execution I have seen musketeers do on schedule of battle, however they discharged at incredible regiments and those additionally sensible near.

But as per Defoe, Irish marksmanship was surprisingly more terrible. 'I guess it won't handily be failed to remember how at the Battel of Agrim, a Battalion of the English Army receiv'd the entire discharge of an Irish Regiment of Dragoons, yet they never knew right up 'til the present time whether they had any Bullets or no.' In Defoe's viewpoint this was basically the aftereffect of absence of training and he needed to see young people surrendering the 'stupid Boyish Sports of Cocking and Cricketing' to focus on shooting.

All in all it is not really shocking that until the finish of the seventeenth century when prior guns were supplanted by the fusil accordingly the term fusilier

— there were some tactical scholars who contended that the flintlock should give way to a weapon which was, they accepted, far prevalent: the longbow.

he musketeer wore no protection. 'The protective arms of a musketeer is a decent boldness', composed General Monck. Yet, this by itself didn't do the trick to beat

off a cavalry charge, and for this reason it was important to consolidate with the other arm of the infantry: the pikeman. A square of pikemen was encircled by two positions of musketeers, the front position stooping. The adversary rangers was permitted to approach, inside twenty yards or something like that, then, at that point, the musketeers terminated, focusing on the ponies' legs. On the off chance that the rangers came on they ended up facing a line of pikes projecting past the two positions of musketeers.

The pikeman was equipped with a blade and a pike, the last sixteen feet in length. He for the most part wore a corselet (a bosom and backplate) and a cap. Contrasted and the musketeer he was an unwieldy figure, and on long summer walks his arms and shield appeared to be oppressive. His absence of versatility some of the time prompted him being abandoned, as when Charles made his night retreat from Oxford in June 1644. Having 'hung lit matches at the factory and extension at Islip' he took with him just his rangers and musketeers. Hence even the pikemen tended increasingly more to leave off body shield. Pikemen stayed a fundamental piece of English militaries all through the seventeenth century and delivered great assistance in protection as well as in assault also. While contradicting armed forces came to tight situation the musketeers terminated a couple of volleys, then, at that point, the pikemen evened out their pikes and charged home. This is the thing that contemporary scholars implied by the expression 'at push of pike', and it was much of the time the definitive second in battle.

ut for Cromwell, obviously, it was the rangers which truly counted. When in 1643, the 'single men and house keepers' of Norwich brought £240 up in request to prepare an organization of foot, Cromwell kept in touch with them, 'I support the business; just I want to prompt you that your foot organization might be transformed into a group of pony; which to be sure will (by God's favoring) undeniably more benefit the reason than a few foot organizations'. Cromwell's recommendation was taken, and the soldiers of pony subsequently raised were prevalently known as 'the Virgin troop', to pay tribute to the youngsters and ladies who had financed it.

Like a large portion of the mounted force of the day they were called harquebusiers, however at this point just officials were furnished with the flintlock harquebus. The troopers typically conveyed only a sword and a couple of guns. They wore bosom and back reinforcement and an iron headpiece, informally known as a 'pot'. Among the mounted force too there was a developing propensity to leave off defensive layer, and absolutely the full suit of shield — the cuirass — was right outdated. 'It will kill a man to serve in an entire cuirass', composed Sir Edmund Verney. However, a couple, who could find ponies sufficiently able to bear the weight,

still attempted it. A regiment of them did great help for Parliament in 1643 and 1644. Being completely covered by a splendid iron shell they were known as 'the regiment of lobsters'.

t the start of the Civil War not many Englishmen knew about the developments of Gustavus Adolphus, and the Dutch arrangement of rangers strategies was as yet standard. This implied running forward in arrangements five or six positions profound, until close enough for each rank thusly to discharge its guns at the foe and afterward ride round to the back. Not until their projectiles had adequately diminished the positions of the adversary did the mounted force plunge to hand to hand battling. Against the more noteworthy capability of black powder guns this move, known as the caracole, sentenced the rangers to ineffectiveness.

furthermore most militaries incorporated a regiment of dragoons, mounted musketeers. During a development they were sent on ahead to get passes and scaffolds until the infantry could come up; during a retreat they remained behind to cover the military's withdrawal. Since they battled by walking, behind supports or in ditches, they could manage with a lot less expensive ponies than the cavalryman. In a Restoration play three worn out musketeers were blamed for transforming themselves into dragooners 'by pillaging a malt-factory of three visually impaired ponies'. Typical fight practice was for one dragoon in ten to stay behind the terminating line and take care of their nags.

Most fights opened with a barrage, however ordnance generally had just a little influence in the remainder of the battle. In any case, inferable from their imperative job in attacks, no military could bear to be without a pony drawn cannons train, and to lose all or a piece of his ordnance was perhaps the most embarrassing thing that could happen to an authority. Definitely the lumbering train seriously restricted a military's versatility, however in December 1643 Sir William Waller had the option to dispatch an effective treat assault on the town of Alton when his gunnery showed up there following a night walk along sloppy paths which were believed to be blocked. His lord heavy armament specialist, Colonel Wemyss, had gotten firearms made of slim metal bound with cowhide. These light calfskin weapons could be pulled by a solitary pony, while a medium field firearm of customary plan required eight or twelve ponies or bulls. It was by such tricks as this that Waller obtained his moniker of the Night Owl.

There was, obviously, significantly more to battle than fights and attacks. 'A military is a monster that hath an extraordinary tummy and should be taken care of.' It was said to describe the Cromwellian missions in Ireland and Scotland that the two nations 'were vanquished by ideal arrangements of Cheshire cheddar and roll'. Yet, at the

start of the Civil War the stock of arrangements was not really efficient. At the point when the Parliamentarian armed force walked to the help of Gloucester it drove alongside it around 1,000 sheep and sixty head of steers, however lamentably lost a significant number of them over the span of battling. Without even a trace of a legitimate commissariat, the act of 'free quarter' was broadly taken on. Householders were obliged to give food and housing to a specific number of troopers and their ponies as a trade-off for a ticket promising installment sometime in the future. Normally the framework was disliked. 'My home,' kept in touch with one lamentable householder, 'is, and hath been brimming with officers this fortnight, such uncivil consumers and parched spirits that a barrel of good lager shakes at seeing them, and the entire house is only a meeting of tobacco and spitting.'

Whenever there was any chance of adversary activity the troopers must be quartered near one another, prepared for moment preparation. Since it was not feasible for the assets of the quick area to be sufficient to take care of so enormous a deluge of populace for over a little while, it was not unexpected important to spread the heap by demanding supplies from a lot more extensive region. As far as anyone knows partnered authorities now and again fought with one another over the size of their individual stockpile regions. It was a framework which was clearly totally open to mishandle. 'Know,' composed the Royalist legislative leader of Worcester, 'that except if you bring to time the month to month commitment, you are to anticipate an unsanctified group of pony among you, from whom in case you conceal yourselves, they will fire your homes without kindness, hang up your bodies any place they track down them, and alarm your phantoms.' Efforts were made to control these maltreatments, since any process for residing off neighborhood assets worked much better in a climate of kindness. As indicated by Clarendon individuals of the Edgehill area were so threatening to the Royalists that 'they diverted or concealed every one of their arrangements, since that there was neither meat for man or pony' and a few fighters had 'scant eaten bread' in the 48 hours before the fight. Not all over the place, obviously, was adequately crowded or rich to have the option to oblige the requirements of a military. In February 1645, when a military was requested to go from Portsmouth to the alleviation of Weymouth, the men needed to require four days' arrangement with them, 'by reason the nations into which they were to go were squandered to the point that they resembled a wild'. The more extended the conflict continued, the more genuine this issue became. By 1645 the sufferings of the populace were to such an extent that in certain spaces they had united together in sporadic militaries to oppose the

requests made by the two sides. Being ineffectively equipped they were known as 'Clubmen'. His dealings with the Clubmen just affirmed Cromwell's conviction that the nation would not pardon him and his kindred administrators and lawmakers in case they neglected to carry the conflict to a quick end.

n such conditions, and especially in Ireland and Scotland, the troopers needed to depend predominantly on what they could convey in their rucksacks. The standard every day proportion per man was 2 lb of bread, 1 lb of meat or (all the more generally) cheddar and a jug of wine or two jugs of brew. At this date drinking water was one certain method of turning out to be sick. Practically speaking, obviously, the warrior was fortunate on the off chance that he got half of his day by day apportion. Obviously his eating regimen probably had some impact on his proficiency, not such a huge amount in the energy of the fight as during the daily practice of the walk. Seventeenth-century armed forces moved at a normal speed of around ten miles per day, which is impressively more slow than the walking pace of 20th century troopers. Among the purposes behind this — helpless streets, awkward gear to convey — we ought to maybe consider the conventional warrior's low day by day admission of calories and protein.

Besides food, the officer required his compensation; frequently he really wanted it to purchase food in the voyaging market which continued in the back of the military. However, in all nations the warrior's compensation was typically falling behind financially. A few authorities accepted that it was useful for discipline in case they kept their fighters somewhat shy of pay. This was called 'taking care of them with trust'. However, assuming their compensation dropped excessively far behind, trust was probably going to go to surrender, and the outcome was departure or insurrection. Toward the beginning of the Civil War the arrangement of armed force finance was in disarray. In April 1643 the Earl of Essex took the field with 16,000 foot and 3000 pony: by July his officials felt obliged to make the accompanying report: 'The quantity of Foot are 3000 walking Men, and somewhere around 3000 debilitated, occasioned by the Want of Pay, sick Cloathing, and any remaining Miseries which go to a neglected wiped out Army'. Assuming these figures are right, above and beyond a large portion of the infantry had abandoned inside 90 days, as an immediate aftereffect of what Essex himself called 'the crying need of the eager officers'. Essex's cavalry held out better; there were as yet 2500 of them. However at that point regardless of whether he accept his compensation — at 2s every day it was, regardless, multiple times that of an infantryman — the mounted force trooper was better ready to care for himself; his ownership of a pony gave him a chose advantage when it came, as it oftentimes did, to looting. In addition it empowered him, when crushed, to escape the field of fight, while poor people trooper was taken prisoner or

butchered where he stood. Consequently the Civil War mounted force were all volunteers. They were for the most part better taught and of higher social remaining than the infantry. They started to lead the pack in generally political and strict developments inside the military. Then again simply by turning to impressment was it conceivable to keep the infantry up to the numbers required. In every town the occupation of impressment was given to the constable and the helpless man endured in side-effect a lot of misuse and provocation; at Upwell in Cambridgeshire the constable was charmed for setting out to intrigue the nearby sorceress' child. Definitely, notwithstanding, the pace of abandonment kept on leftover high among squeezed men who were paid just a worker's pay, 8d every day, and that irregularly.

It isn't difficult to see the reason why, as per Sir Ralph Hopton, the aphorism of a decent broad was 'Compensate fairly, order well and hang well'. Cromwell's letters — like those of different authorities — are brimming with demands for cash to pay his soldiers, and right from the beginning still up in the air to keep great discipline. In April 1643 a paper announced that 'the Colonel [i.e. Cromwell] practices severe discipline, for when two troopers would have escapt, he sent for them back, made them be whipt at the commercial center in Huntingdon, and ... turned them off as rebels'. Among different disciplines utilized were riding the wooden pony for minor offenses, drilling through the tongue with an intensely hot iron for profanation, and going through the test of endurance for burglary. In pretty much all of his missions Cromwell balanced a couple of men as marauders. Without a doubt harsh measures were required. Remarking on the indiscipline of the Parliamentary armed force in the early months of the conflict, John Hampden composed 'in case this go on for a spell, the military will develop as accursed to the nation as the Cavaliers'. To stay away from this, one Roundhead troop when they went pillaging claimed to be Cavaliers.

In time Cromwell's and Fairfax's soldiers became popular for their appropriate conduct. 'I recollect,' composed Sir Philip Warwick, 'what a calm companion of mine let me know that he answered to an old associate of his drew in with Fairfax vaunting the sacredness of their military and the carelessness of our own. "Confidence", says he, "thou sayest valid; for in our military we have the transgressions of men [drinking and wenching] yet in yours you have those of fallen angels, otherworldly pride and disobedience".' There is a bit of common pride about the expression 'sins of men' which accords well with the engraving on the norm of one Cavalier regiment: 'Cuckolds we come'. Among the 'wrongdoings of demons' should be counted an overabundance of moral resentment. The Battle of Naseby finished in the

slaughter of something like 100 of the ones who continued in the caravan — the leaguer — behind the Royalist armed force. There were a few hundred of these 'leaguer bitches' at Naseby, and the individuals who were not killed were set apart out as prostitutes by having their countenances sliced or their noses cut. Not that the sexual requirements of the Royalist fighters had been provided food for with the expert productivity normal for the mainland armed forces. Eight prostitutes for every hundred troopers was the suggested proportion in the Spanish powers, while one power, writing in 1617, determined that there were more than 4000 'prostitutes, young men and off color carts' to 3000 German officers. Via contrast a prostitute observed after the Scottish armed force should be hanged assuming she were at that point wedded, while in case she were single the executioner was to wed her without a moment's delay (apparently to the man she was found with) and afterward scourge her out of the military. It isn't difficult to see the reason why Charles II never felt calm in Scotland.

It isn't at all unmistakable what occurred in the Parliamentary militaries. Contemporary melody writing gives the feeling that ladies who wished to follow the Roundheads had as a matter of first importance to camouflage themselves, Polly Oliver design, as warriors — however in one such case, a promising military vocation was hindered by the introduction of a youthful officer. Cromwell's men were not altogether without human frailties, be that as it may. On one well known event, in January 1646, they dispatched an unexpected assault on the base camp of a little Royalist armed force. They raged the house and burst into a room where the clueless Royalist officials were partaking in a round of cards. In any case, with particular sound judgment the Royalists tossed the stake-cash out of a window; Cromwell's soldiers jumped out after it, and the Royalists got away through the back door.

4. A Lovely Company

ON 29 August 1642, only seven days in the wake of King Charles increased his expectation at Nottingham, Cromwell summoned his group of pony at Huntingdon. Indeed, even in these little beginnings Cromwell's speed and conclusiveness of activity is obvious. A fortnight later he was requested to join the really Parliamentary armed force under the Earl of Essex at Northampton. The Earl had some experience of battle on the mainland — however very little, and he had minimal normal ability. In any case, he was a baron and he was absolutely solid; these two characteristics counted for a lot, particularly when the faithfulness of numerous men was questionable — 'they will go with the tide' as Lord Willoughby composed. However, not the strong, pipe-smoking Earl of Essex. Had he been crushed he may well have been attempted and executed for treachery; yet he was prepared amazing the reason. At the point when he did battle he took with him his casket and winding sheet.

Cromwell's troop was placed into Essex's own regiment of pony thus partook in the Battle of Edgehill on 23 October. In this fight two unpracticed militaries conflicted and the outcome was absolute disorder. Neither side truly realized what was occurring nor who had won — however normally both professed to have acquired a triumph. Ruler Charles, it is valid, was left in charge of the field of fight and he was allowed to walk on towards London — yet he had been allowed to do that before the fight at any rate. By 12 November he had progressed similar to Brentford, yet the following day he was checked by the London prepared groups drawn up at Turnham Green. Cromwell's own part in the Edgehill and Turnham Green missions remains covered in haziness. At Edgehill it appears to be that he showed up after the expected time in the day — without a doubt he was subsequently blamed for intentionally keeping away from the front line out and out. As per Sir William Dugdale he had gone up into a congregation steeple to review the scene with his 'point of view glass' (for example telescope). On seeing the defeat of the Parliamentary rangers he concluded that carefulness was the better piece of boldness and 'made such hast to be gone, that as opposed to sliding the steps by which he came up, he swing'd down the Bell-rope and fled with his troop'. In any case, whatever Cromwell might have done that day everything in his later profession clarifies that he was not a coward.

Though his own part in the fight was most likely concise and may have been shameful, Edgehill was to profoundly affect Cromwell's reasoning. On the Royalist side Prince Rupert had demanded that everything be done in the advanced Swedish style. This might have done close to confound the evil

prepared Royalist infantry, however there can be no question that it was to reform mounted force fighting in England. Gustavus Adolphus had drawn up his mounted force in just three positions and trained them to charge directly into the foe lines, maintaining close control, and saving their fire as late as possible, then, at that point, laying about them with the blade. By embracing these strategies at Edgehill against rivals still married to the antiquated Dutch techniques, Rupert's cavalry scored a staggering achievement. Cromwell was intrigued and from that point on was to duplicate Rupert at whatever point he got the opportunity. Yet, it was not simply an issue of strategies. The Royalist cavalry were for the most part refined men, acquainted with going hunting riding a horse. After Edgehill Cromwell examined the fight with John Hampden and numerous years after the fact he reviewed this conversation.

At my first going into this commitment I saw our men were beaten at each hand … and I wanted him that he would make increments … of some new regiments; and I let him know I would be functional to him in bringing such men as I suspected had a soul that would accomplish something in the work. 'Your troopers,' said I, 'are the greater part of them old rotted servingmen and tapsters and such sort of colleagues; and,' said I, 'their troopers are noble men's children, more youthful children and people of value; do you believe that the spirits of such base and mean colleagues will be ever ready to experience respectable men that have honor and mental fortitude and goal in them? You should get men of a soul that is probably going to happen the extent that refined men will do, or, more than likely you will be beaten still.' He [Hampden] was a savvy and commendable individual; and he imagined that I talked a decent thought yet an unrealistic one. Genuinely I let him know I could do to some degree in it. I did as such … I raised such men as had the dread of God before them, as made some heart of what they did, and from that day forward … they were never beaten.

In the mid year of 1642 Cromwell had gotten Cambridgeshire for the

Parliamentary reason, however Cambridgeshire couldn't battle the King all alone; the conflict, to be pursued adequately, must be pursued on a more extensive material. As ahead of schedule as July of that year Parliament had perceived that co-activity between nearby provinces was fundamental, however this ideal was in no way, shape or form simple to accomplish. The country upper class framed nearby tribes; regularly enthusiastically dedicated to the interests of their own gathering — the local area of the shire — they just seldom and hesitantly looked past its boundaries. At the point when Cromwell's companions and neighbors utilized the words 'my country', they didn't mean England; they implied Cambridgeshire or Huntingdonshire. However a conflict against the King couldn't be directed by various separate districts, each going its own

way, raising its own military and arranging its own mission. Some type of affiliation, some sort of military and political partnership between a square of regions was plainly and earnestly required, however taking into account the instilled parochialism of the country upper class it could scarcely be an unconstrained development. To set up such an affiliation would require difficult work and consideration, even more so since its general purpose was to plan for war, and this was a disturbing and cash devouring strategy which most citizens would have liked to see delayed endlessly. In the present circumstance the drive needed to come from the centre.

On 20 December 1642 Parliament passed a statute for the combination of five provinces: Norfolk, Suffolk, Cambridgeshire, Hertfordshire and Essex, under the general order of Lord Gray of Warke. In any case, the neighborhood nobility were not in such a rush as the 'strong and grisly disapproved of men' who sat at Westminster and for quite a long time the Eastern Association existed distinctly on paper. In mid-January 1643 Cromwell drove a group of pony from London to Cambridge. In transit he halted at St Albans to capture the Royalist sheriff of Hertfordshire — no simple assignment since the sheriff had the help of a commercial center group and twenty furnished troopers must be sent in to grab him from their defensive consideration. Once at Cambridge Cromwell started to make some waves. The letters he composed right now uncover a desire to move quickly which still up in the air to convey to others.

We intreat that you would make all conceivable speed to have in status, against any notification will be given, a significant power of Horse and Foot to get together with us, to hold any foe's power back from breaking in upon your yet peaceable country. For we have specific knowledge that some of

Prince Rupert's powers are come similar to Wellingborough in Northamptonshire, and that the Papists in Norfolk are requested to rise by and by upon you.

nder the strain of this 'certain insight' the area councils of Cambridgeshire, Suffolk, Norfolk and Essex organized a joint gathering at Bury on 9 February. Progressively the Eastern Association started to come to fruition. In April the joint gatherings were changed into a long-lasting organization by the foundation of the Cambridge Committee: two individuals from every one of the five provinces and one from the City of Norwich. The advisory group before long ran into monetary troubles and thought that it is difficult to practice a lot of power over the constituent districts, however somewhere around a beginning had been made in the assignment of furnishing the Association with the foundation of a focal administration.

Throughout the spring of 1643 Cromwell locked in to the work of

invigorating and posting Cambridge. He was currently a colonel and hence compelled by a solemn obligation to raise and prepare an entire regiment. By March he had five soldiers; by September ten; and by mid 1644 fourteen — however the typical number of troops in a regiment was just six. However, definitely more than simple numbers it was the nature of his officers that counted. 'A couple of legit men,' he composed, 'are superior to numbers.' His selecting strategy was depicted by perhaps the most well known seventeenth-century Puritan, Richard Baxter.

At his initial entry into the conflicts, being nevertheless a commander of pony, he had uncommon consideration to get strict men into his troop. These men were of more prominent comprehension than normal fighters, and in this way were fearful of the significance and result of war ... he that taketh the felicity of Church and State to be his end, esteemeth it over his life, and thusly will the sooner set out his life for it. Also men of parts and understanding expertise to deal with this business, and realize that flying is the surest way to no end, and that remaining to it is the likeliest method for getting away, there being numerous normally that fall in trip for one that falls in fearless battle ... These things 'tis plausible Cromwell comprehended; and that none would be such drawn in brave men as the strict. Yet, yet I guess, that at his initially picking such men into his troop, it was the very regard and love of strict men that basically moved him; and the keeping away from of those issues, mutinous plunderings and complaints of the nation ... which the degraded in militaries are normally at real fault for. By this implies he for sure sped better compared to he expected ... that troop demonstrated so bold, that to the furthest extent that I could learn they not even once fled before an enemy.

Baxter was a moderate Puritan who opposed unequivocally of a portion of the more extreme strict developments which were to create inside the military. In 1643 he was offered the chaplaincy of Cromwell's regiment, yet declined it

— a choice he was to lament. A long time later he composed that 'these very men that welcomed me to be their minister, were the men that subsequently headed a large part of the military and some of them were the forwardest in the entirety of our changes; which made me wish I had gone among them ... for then all the fire was in one spark'.It is evident that one outcome of Cromwell's assurance to enroll strict men who were focused on the reason was that he was ready to pick as officials men of a lower social remaining than the majority of his counterparts thought appropriate. In 1645 the Earl of Manchester grumbled that Cromwell didn't pick 'men of domain, however, for example, were normal men,

poor and of mean parentage, just he would provide them with the title of faithful, valuable men ... assuming you view his own regiment of pony, see what a multitude there is of those that call themselves genuine; some of them proclaim they have seen dreams and had disclosures'. As Cromwell himself put it, while guarding the decision of Ralph Margery as chief of his thirteenth troop, 'I had rather have a plain reddish brown covered skipper that knows what he battles for, and loves what he knows, than that which you call a courteous fellow and isn't anything else', and later, 'It had been well that praiseworthy people and birth had gone into these occupations, however for what reason do they not show up? Who might have frustrated them? In any case, seeing it was so vital the work should continue, preferred plain men over none ... various plain, faithful men like John Lilburne passed on their situations in Essex's military to find a more amicable home in the Eastern Association.

Cromwell's first assignment was to shield the Association against both inner and outside foes. On 14 March Parliament requested him to manage an undermined Royalist ascending at Lowestoft — however it had been done even before these directions can have contacted him. His five soldiers left Cambridge on Sunday 12 March. Following day they 'visited' some Royalist houses close to Norwich. On Wednesday, helped by volunteers from Norwich and Yarmouth, they walked to Lowestoft. They observed the street covered by a battery of three firearms and a chain attracted across it to keep out the mounted force. Cromwell called upon the town to give up. Gravely misjudging the strength of their position the Royalists rejected. Cromwell sent in a party of dragoons. They got off, slithered under the chain and progressed upon the firearms, waving their guns menacingly. It was adequate. The protectors escaped; the chain was broken and the troopers rode in. They held onto a store of arms and captured the main Royalists. One man, Sir John Wentworth, consented to give £1000 to Cromwell's conflict depository to have his offense disregarded. In the wake of expenditure two productive days in Lowestoft, Cromwell got back to Norwich where he stayed until the evening of 19 March. Then, at that point, by riding the entire evening, he entered King's Lynn right off the bat Monday morning, seized and incapacitated known Royalist supporters and caught a little boat with a freight of arms from Dunkirk. By Wednesday, following a bustling ten days, he was back in Cambridge. It was generally valuable exercise for his quickly developing regiment of horse.

On 7 April Lord Gray for certain 5000 men, the greater part of the Association's powers, passed on Cambridge to join the super Parliamentary armed force at the attack of

Reading. Cromwell was abandoned in charge of a little separation liable for the safeguard of the Association's north-west outskirts. The central danger came from the Newark Royalists whose lightning attacks into Lincolnshire had caused frustration all through the entire of the Fen Country. Cromwell moved his soldiers to Huntingdon and sent a post of dragoons to Wisbech. He chose to hang tight of the Ouse and mentioned the related regions to track down the cash to sustain its extensions. However at that point, seeing that the Newarkers were occupied by occasions somewhere else, Cromwell headed toward the assault. On 22 April he involved Peterborough, where his troopers scoured the basilica. On the twenty-fifth he laid attack to Crowland, an unassuming community all around shielded both naturally and by one of Cromwell's Royalist cousins. The underlying attack was thumped back, yet notwithstanding the inconveniences of a Fenland attack in wet and breezy climate, Cromwell's men adhered to it for three days, in length enough for the safeguards to lose heart and give up. These increases empowered the Association — destined to be fortified by the expansion of Huntingdonshire — to utilize the River Nene as its boondocks, consequently making it essentially invulnerable to assault from the north. While in this space Cromwell visited his uncle, Sir Oliver, who had resigned to Ramsey after the offer of Hinchingbroke. Since Sir Oliver was a Royalist he held onto his arms and plate, and yet remembered to doff his cap in the elderly person's presence.

These nearby victories implied that Cromwell was called upon to act inside the system of a more extensive procedure — and to be made always persuasively mindful of the troubles engaged with convincing neighborhood administrators to co-work successfully. The Lord General, the Earl of Essex, had gotten knowledge that a caravan of ammo was in transit from the north to Oxford. He requested Lord Gray of Groby, the officer of the East Midlands Association, to join powers with Cromwell and with the Lincolnshire Parliamentarians, under Lord Willoughby and John Hotham, to keep this imperative escort from breaking through to the King. The arranged interference won't ever appear. The guard arrived at Oxford securely, its escort looting Leicestershire and Northamptonshire on the way. Cromwell accused Lord Gray, while the Lincolnshire advisory group accused every other person (counting Cromwell). Not until 9 May did Cromwell and the Lincolnshire troops — however not Lord Gray — rendezvous at Sleaford, on the Lincoln—Peterborough street. By then it was past the point of no return. Yet, for all that the occasions of the following not many days were to be critical throughout the entire existence of Cromwell's

military profession. Moving gradually westwards the joined powers ran over a foe power two miles outside Grantham late in the evening of 13 May. For thirty minutes the different sides traded flintlock fire. Then, at that point, seeing that the Royalists were hesitant to propel, Cromwell and his kindred authorities chose finally to step up to the plate. 'We came on with our soldiers a really round jog, they standing firm to get us; and our men charging furiously upon them, by God's fortune they were promptly directed, and fled, and we had the execution of them a few miles.' Thus, for a minor scope, Cromwell had demonstrated to himself and to his men that he could do what Rupert had done at Edgehill. The Lincolnshire troops, notwithstanding, had performed perceptibly less well thus it was chosen to resign to Lincoln.

The consolidated power was soon in real life once more. Master Fairfax and his child, Sir Thomas Fairfax, required assistance if they somehow managed to follow up Sir Thomas' triumph at Wakefield on 21 May. This time Lords Gray and Willoughby, John Hotham and Cromwell prevailed with regards to collecting a significant armed force — around 6000 men — at Nottingham toward the month's end. Yet, nothing happened to the projected walk north. While there was as yet a functioning Cavalier power at Newark neither the Lincolnshire men nor the East Midlanders were ready to cross the Humber. Subsequently the Fairfaxes were steered by Newcastle's mind-boggling numbers at the Battle of Adwalton Moor on 3o June.

meanwhile the military at Nottingham had been given another errand. They were to be prepared to dispatch a diversionary strike on Oxford in case of the

Earl of Essex moving south. Yet, any desire for them doing this task was broken by the squabble between John Hotham and different authorities. At the point when they grumbled about the evil discipline of the Lincolnshire troops his answer was that he battled for freedom and expected to appreciate it no matter what. During a disagreement regarding oats he turned his cannon on Cromwell. Hotham's conduct prompted questions about his dependability to the reason. He was watched and was found to be in steady correspondence with the Cavaliers at Newark. On 18 June Hotham was captured by Sir John Meldrum, an expert officer whom Essex had shipped off assume in general responsibility for the powers at Nottingham. He got away, nonetheless, and escaped to Lincoln. From that point he kept in touch with the Speaker of the House fighting his honesty and demanding that he had been badly utilized by Cromwell and his officials. In his view they were upstarts with hazardously extreme sentiments. 'The courage of these men had just yet showed up in their mutilating of holy places.' Eventually he was re-captured at Hull while he was attempting to

organize its acquiescence to the Queen. Because of Hotham's abandonment the Nottingham armed force deteriorated. The Lincolnshire troops had headed out with their authority and different contingents before long followed. Subsequently a subsequent weapons escort, and the Queen herself, broke securely through to Oxford.

In each quarter the conflict was going severely for Parliament. In the south west Sir Ralph Hopton and his Cornish infantry were winning triumph after triumph for the Royalist cause. The north was overwhelmed by the military raised by the Earl of Newcastle. In the middle the King had set up his central command at Oxford and in the battling among Reading and Oxford, John Hampden was killed. On 26 July 1643, Rupert surprised Bristol, in this manner giving the Royalists a crucial place for the import and assembling of arms. Both Hopton and Newcastle worked freely of the King; he had no compelling command over them and hence there could be no doubt of a Royalist Grand Strategy. There was no arrangement for a three-pronged assault on London in 1643. In any case on all fronts the Royalists were progressing admirably, while an excessive number of the Parliamentary administrators were fixated by the requirements of neighborhood defence.

Throughout these occasions Cromwell had been a backer of a more versatile armed force — a 'running' or a 'flying armed force' as it was called — and of a more extended scope of procedure. However at that point he was fortunate. As he, at the end of the day, brought up in a letter written in June 1643, the Eastern Association's regular stream and fen safeguards were solid; the heft of its powers could securely be utilized away from home. The administrators in Lincolnshire and the Midlands didn't enjoy this valuable benefit thus, contrasted and Cromwell, they regularly show up in a troublesome light, over-mindful and obstructionist. Not, obviously, that Cromwell's men were resistant from the overall hesitance to travel. Renunciation from his powers was attributed by the Cambridge board to the 'eronious assessment of our unpracticed nation fighters that they should not to be drawne or ledd past the limits of the fyve districts'. Yet, Cromwell's principle issue was, definitely, a monetary one. Where could he observe the cash to pay his men before they pawned their weapons and returned home? The majority of his letters return over and over to this theme.

I entreat you, rush the stock to us; fail to remember not cash. I press not hard, however I do as such need that, I guarantee you, the foot and the dragooners are prepared to revolt. Lay not all that much upon the rear of a helpless noble man, who wants, absent a lot of commotion, to set out his life, and drain the last drop to serve the Cause and you. I ask not your cash for myself, in case that were my end and hope

(viz. the compensation of my place), I would not open my mouth right now. I want to deny myself; yet others won't be fulfilled. I implore you hurry supplies.

Initially the cash for raising and keeping up with Cromwell's soldiers, similar to the remainder of the Association's powers, came from deliberate commitments. Partially this was on the grounds that Parliament would have rather not see any of its income from tax assessment redirected from Essex's principle armed force and to a limited extent since men trusted that the conflict would before long be finished. In March 1643 Cromwell composed hopefully 'one month's compensation might demonstrate all your difficulty'. However, the impact of this framework was to toss all the weight on the shoulders of a couple of sharp Parliamentarians while the people who were tepid or impassive got away softly. In May, after much pushing from the Cambridge board of trustees, the House of Commons passed the Ordinance of the Fifth and Twentieth empowering the Association to address its issues through neighborhood appraisal and tax collection. By pre-fall this new framework was in full swing.

In mid-July the Earl of Essex requested Meldrum and Cromwell to meet him at Stony Stratford to get ready for an assault on Oxford. However, presently it was Cromwell's chance to feel, and submit to, the tension of neighborhood needs. The Newark Cavaliers had held onto Stamford and were progressing towards Peterborough. Of itself this was not an intense danger to the Association's outskirts protections; as Cromwell would like to think a few hundred men could hang tight. What was disturbing, nonetheless, was the news that the Earl of Newcastle's military was on the walk, and may before long overwhelm the little power with which Lord Willoughby was holding Gainsborough. Without a moment's delay Meldrum turned north, towards Gainsborough, while Cromwell got the Cavaliers out of Stamford, giving them no an ideal opportunity to brace the town. They withdrew to a close by chateau, Burghley House, the home of the Earl of Exeter, and were adequately certain to dismiss Cromwell's proposal of terms. On 24 July, after a short cannons assault, Cromwell requested his musketeers to storm the house. As they broke in, the Cavaliers, seeing that everything was lost, concluded that they would, all things considered, really like to be conceded quarter and Cromwell was sufficiently liberal to give it them. Sending a few hundred detainees to Cambridge he then, at that point, rushed on with his cavalry to find Meldrum. They met a Lincolnshire power at a meeting at North Scarle on 27 July.

t 2 a.m. following day they moved off toward Gainsborough where Willoughby was attacked by Newcastle's more youthful sibling, Lord Cavendish. In the van of the calming armed force rode the Lincolnshire troops, then, at that point, came the Midlanders, while Cromwell's regiment raised the back — in all twenty

soldiers of pony and four of dragoons. As they moved toward the town Cavendish drew up his men on a precarious slope neglecting the street. Notwithstanding the strength of the foe's position Cromwell and his kindred administrators had no real option except to assault it, or pass on Willoughby to his destiny. The Lincolnshire men drove an energize the slope, dismissing some resistance. Once at the top they attempted to get into fight request, yet what with the disarray of the rising and the troublesome ground — it was studded with bunny openings — they were as yet in confusion when the fundamental body of the foe progressed towards them. With Cromwell now in charge of the traditional they met this development with their very own charge. Along these lines, as would be natural for Cromwell, 'we came up pony to horse, where we questioned it with our swords and guns a lovely time, all maintaining close control, so nobody could break the other'. In the long run, notwithstanding, the Royalists started to give ground. Immediately the strain on them was expanded until they turned in flight and were sought after for five miles or thereabouts. Be that as it may, Cavendish had kept one regiment for possible later use and with this he assaulted the four

Lincolnshire troops which had not participated in the joy of the pursuit. Cromwell himself appears to have been among the followers, however this didn't keep him from seeing what was occurring. Seeing was a certain something, taking care of business, another. The cavalry officer has no harder undertaking than controlling a charge whenever it has been dispatched. Rupert had been not able to do this at Edgehill and, subsequently, had not returned on schedule to take further part in the fight. In any case, this is exactly what Cromwell presently figured out how to do. With the assistance of Major Whalley, and 'with much ado' — these three little words show up in the account letter composed by the officials in charge of the Lincolnshire powers — he prevailed with regards to recovering command north of three of his soldiers. They rushed back to the location of the activity where Cavendish's save seemed to have won the day. What occurred there can best be left in Cromwell's own words.

promptly fell upon his back with my three soldiers, who did as such astound him, that he gave over the pursuit [of the Lincolnshire troops] and would fain have conveyed himself from me, however I pushing on constrained them down a slope, having great execution of them, and underneath the slope, drove the General [Cavendish] with a portion of his fighters into a mess, where my skipper lieutenant slew him with a push under his short ribs.

The victors then, at that point, set with regards to the occupation of sending supplies of ammo and powder into Gainsborough fully expecting the recharged attack it would need to suffer when Newcastle's principle armed force came up. However, the jubilant

leaders were in for a terrible shock. Here, by and by, are Cromwell's words.

ord was presented to us that the adversary had around six soldiers of pony, and 300 foot, a little on the opposite side of the town. Upon this we coaxed musketeers out of the town and with our assortment of pony walked towards them. We saw two soldiers towards the plant, which my men crashed down into a little town at the lower part of the slope. At the point when we accompanied our pony to the highest point of that slope we found in the last an entire regiment of foot, after that undeniably an and, as some counted, around fifty shades of foot, with an extraordinary collection of horse.

Newcastle's military was at that point there. Splendid as Cromwell's activity at Gainsborough had been, it had arrived too behind schedule to save the town.

Worse still the soothing armed force was itself now at risk for being obliterated. The foot withdrew, in frenzy and turmoil, back into

Gainsborough, where they were comparable to lost. Cromwell had no real option except to return as fast as conceivable to Lincoln — no simple assignment when the two his men and ponies were depleted after the day's battling and were gone against by new powers in overpowering strength. However they oversaw it. Four soldiers of Cromwell's regiment under Major Whalley and four Lincoln troops under Captain Ayscough took it in goes to stand and face the adversary to cover the retreat of the fundamental body. On eight or nine separate events a small bunch of men held the Royalists under control while their companions pulled out to security. It was greatly done, without misfortune, a retreat, as Cromwell composed 'equivalent to any of late occasions, and its honor had a place with Major Whalley and Captain Ayscough, next under God'. Deliberately the activity at Gainsborough had accomplished nothing. The entire of Lincolnshire was before long lost and Cromwell himself pulled out to Peterborough and Spalding, wanting to hang tight of the Nene. Be that as it may, as far as Cromwell's own profession its importance is this. With under a year's experience of war he had effectively shown that he could dominate the two hardest issues confronting a cavalry commandant: how to keep control of a fruitful charge, and how to withdraw when in a miserable circumstance. Two things made this conceivable. Right off the bat he trained his soldiers to charge at 'a really round run' — though the Cavaliers consistently appear to have been in an over the top rush. Besides the confidence and self-restraint of Cromwell's men was top notch. They could oppose the impulse to pursue loot and obvious targets. 'Really,' composed Cromwell, 'I believe that he who supplicates and lectures best will battle best.' By picking and preparing his own men he accomplished a level of command over his cavalry which no other

pioneer could approach. Ruler Rupert couldn't — his Cavaliers didn't warmly embrace this sort of limitation — while Sir William Waller depicted his pony as 'such miscreants as he would never manage them'.

In the mid year of 1643 the testing opportunity arrived toward the Eastern Association. Its very presence remained in a critical state. In August, in assumption for Newcastle's victorious walk into East Anglia, Royalist components in King's Lynn assumed control over the town. Cromwell multiplied and yet again tried harder to collect men and cash. His letters of this period are brimming with a feeling of emergency. 'It's done questioning, however [get] out quickly everything you can. Raise every one of your groups; send them to Huntingdon; get up what volunteers you can; rush your ponies.' Or once more, 'Ruler Newcastle will progress into your guts; his military is incredible. Better join when others will join and can get together with you, than stay till all be lost; rush to our assistance.' It was during these horrendous weeks that Cromwell started to enroll officials whose low economic wellbeing frightened a portion of the more safe individuals from the neighborhood gentry. The chiefs of his initial five soldiers had all been firmly identified with him by blood or marriage. Presently the opportunity had arrived to dispose of such shows. As he composed, 'You see the need of leaving our old speed.'

Be that as it may, what saved East Anglia was not an unconstrained ascending individuals to ward off the northern gatecrasher, nor was it the expertise of any one officer. It was just the hesitance of Newcastle's soldiers to leave their families a long ways behind, especially when their homes were compromised by trying mounted force attacks drove by Sir Thomas Fairfax, the child of Lord Fairfax, the Parliamentary legislative leader of Hull. So Newcastle turned around north to assault Hull and this gave the hysterical powers of the Eastern Association a breathing space. Cromwell had plainly been frustrated by the reaction of neighborhood specialists to his allures for help. At Westminster men had shown a lot quicker consciousness of the reality of the position. It was right now that the Commons acknowledged the Solemn League and Covenant with the Scots, perceiving that in their frantic circumstance it was important to welcome an unfamiliar armed force into the nation to help them. However, there were many individuals who viewed the cure as being more awful than the infection, among them Lord Gray of Warke whose mentality on this inquiry prompted him being alleviated of the order of the Eastern Association. In his place the Earl of Manchester, once in the past Lord Mandeville, was selected Major-General. By 16 August the Commons had discussed and supported a progression of laws giving him power to raise a huge multitude of both mounted force and infantry. Up to 20,000

troopers could be intrigued in the constituent regions. At long last, by the mandate of 20 September, the Association's military was finally allotted a clear aggregate for its upkeep. The areas, which presently included Lincolnshire, were to find £5630 per week for this purpose.

Cromwell had been named one of Manchester's four Colonels of Horse and he was soon in real life once more, giving a cavalry screen to the Association's infantry which was attacking King's Lynn. With Royalist powers still in strength in Lincolnshire it was a fundamental undertaking, however maybe somewhat uninteresting. Additional intriguing possibilities were opened up by a plan to save Sir Thomas Fairfax's soldiers of pony which were cooped up inside the dividers of Hull by Newcastle's attacking armed force, where they could do nothing but bad. However the arrangement was hazardous, the compensations of accomplishment were extraordinary since this fine rangers general and his regiments would be a most significant expansion to the battling power available to Parliament. Cromwell moved north, first to Boston where Lord Willoughby actually held out with the remainders of the Lincolnshire Parliamentarians. Then, at that point, on 18 September, driving the Royalists before them, Cromwell's development watch arrived at Barton. Fairfax, in the mean time, had been collecting a little armada of boats and he currently carried his 21 soldiers over the Humber as quick as could be expected, crossing with each tide.

When Newcastle found what was occurring he sent new contingents to build up the Lincolnshire Royalists; together they attempted to forestall hero and safeguarded from arriving at the wellbeing of Boston. The specific grouping of occasions is in no way, shape or form clear. The one report of Cromwell's which endures is tantalizingly brief.

The foe quartered inside four miles of us and kept the field the entire night with his entire body. With these he endeavored our watchmen and our quarters, and, assuming that God had not been forgiving, had destroyed us before we had known about it, the five soldiers we set to watch bombing quite a bit of their obligation. However, we got to pony, and withdrew all neat and tidy ... And for this we are incredibly bound to the decency of God, who brought our soldiers off with so little loss.

Obviously something had turned out badly and we realize that Cromwell faulted Lord Willoughby for it; his unexpected had clearly made off without notice the others of the Royalist advance. A few months after the fact Cromwell gave a discourse in the Commons because of which Willoughby was eliminated from his post as Major-General of Lincolnshire and supplanted by the Earl of Manchester. Yet, it might likewise be that different soldiers other than Willoughby's were to blame. En route to the Humber Cromwell sent a letter to his cousin

Oliver St John in which he griped of the nature of a portion of the men under his order. 'A large number of my Lord Manchester's soldiers are come to me: exceptionally awful and mutinous, not to be trusted in,' and he proceeded to balance them with his own regiment. 'I have an exquisite organization; you would regard them, did you know them. They are no Anabaptists, they are straightforward, calm Christians: they hope to be utilized as men.' The undertaking came hazardously near calamity and surprisingly its effective decision was touched with disillusionment. William Harlackenden, the compensation expert of the Essex unexpected, depicted Cromwell's re-visitation of Boston. 'He sobbed when he came to Boston and tracked down no funds for him … he says that he views cash as little as any man, however for his soldiers in case they have not cash expediently they are in a scattered condition.' Despite Cromwell's tears at its end the scene denoted the start of a popular association. Sir Thomas Fairfax, dark looked at and with long dim hair, was twelve years more youthful than Cromwell. He was a bumbling, unobtrusive and profoundly strict man, supposed to be a lot affected by his better half, Lady Anne. However, in the fieriness of fight this peaceful man found inside himself stores of enraged energy; he became, as one contemporary put it, 'changed into an angel'.

Both genders' excellencies were in him
consolidated He had the wildness of the
manliest kind, But all the quietness too of
womankind.

His men cherished him, calling him 'Dark Tom'.

On 7 October, after effectively finishing up the attack of King's Lynn, Manchester raised the infantry to join Cromwell and Fairfax at Boston. From that point they chose to progress to lay attack to Bolingbroke Castle. On 11 October close to the villa of Winceby they experienced a Royalist armed force shipped off alleviate the palace. For once Cromwell prompted against fight, because their mounts were depleted — a trademark illustration of his anxiety for ponies — yet he was overruled by Manchester. Notwithstanding his hesitance, Cromwell was placed in charge of the vanguard. As he drove his cavalry nice and easy the Royalist dragoons set aside opportunity to shoot two volleys at point-dud reach. Cromwell's pony was hit and fell, moving on top of him. Cromwell rose to his feet just to be thumped down again in the mêlée. At last Cromwell was remounted on a 'helpless pony' brought to him by a trooper. Indeed, even without him, nonetheless, his song singing warriors had the option to hold the Royalists until Fairfax chose the day by bringing the second line of rangers round to charge in upon the foe's left flank. Aside from the pursuit it was all over

in 30 minutes. Manchester and Fairfax had won a fine triumph. On the day after Winceby Newcastle raised the attack of Hull and pulled out toward the north. Taking advantage of his lucky break Manchester re-involved the remainder of Lincolnshire. The tide of war was finally starting to turn.

5. The Road to Marston Moor

WITH the beginning of winter came a break in the battling. However, Cromwell was as yet a lawmaker and there was a lot to do at Westminster. In spite of his own triumphs the year overall had been an awful one for Parliament. They had lost more frequently than they had won and right toward the year's end came the most genuine loss of all. John Pym kicked the bucket of disease on 8 December 1643. There had been times when just his political expertise and patient assurance saved Parliament from complete deterioration. None of his replacements in the House of Commons had very his capacity to check and control party difficulty. So particularly far as Manchester and the other armed force administrators were concerned this was a significant issue since they were every one of them hampered by troubles of supply and monetary association — hardships which must be overwhelmed with the assistance of new parliamentary legislation.

In the Eastern Association the £5630 seven days set up by the statute of 20 September was just insufficient to pay and prepare the exceptionally huge armed force which Manchester was raising. As a result the state of a portion of the soldiers came up short; 'no arms, no garments, no tones, no drums — in so bare a stance that to utilize them were to kill them'. Also the heft of the cash was gathered by the singular district panels for the utilization of the soldiers brought up in their own regions; hence the substantial expense of keeping up with Cromwell's regiment was borne by Huntingdonshire alone, by the least fortunate of the constituent areas. Yet, this decentralized framework was not just unjustifiable. It didn't permit mass acquisition of normalized hardware which would have been both less expensive and more productive. It implied the concurrent presence, one next to the other, of a few unique frameworks of bookkeeping and it gave Manchester, at the middle, very little command over his own incomes. Sir William Waller, in a similar situation, discussed his 'acquired powers' which 'having no reliance upon me, however upon them that sent them, would not follow me farther than satisfied themselves, yet would be prepared to walk home when they had sought after their point, as though they had done what's necessary when they had done anything'. In a realistic expression he depicted the multitude of the South Eastern Association as being 'so compounded of city and nation regiments that when they satisfied they may take me to pieces like a clock'. Waller never figured out how to rebuild the design of the South Eastern Association; and this to a great extent clarifies his unremarkable military record in 1644.

Nicknamed William the Conqueror because of his initial victories, this fine broad step by step slipped out of spotlight. The Eastern Association armed force in 1644 was a totally different recommendation. On 20 January 1644 a mandate was passed, expanding the evaluations imposed on the seven areas by 50% and building up a concentrated monetary association. Its section had been smoothed by a perfectly tuned parliamentary mission where Cromwell assumed an essential part. The party divisions inside the Commons had become so sharp and once in a while so unpleasant that it was difficult to get any action through. However, by mollifying a few gatherings and abrogating others by the sheer power and eagerness of his contentions Cromwell guaranteed that the case for transforming the Eastern Association didn't go down in a welter of political interest. On 22 January Cromwell was authorized Lieutenant-General. Prior in the month a Scottish armed force, 21,000 in number, crossed the Tweed. Other than consenting to pay the Scots, Parliament had vowed to change the English church along Scottish Presbyterian lines. Right off the bat in February the Committee of Both Kingdoms (for example Britain and Scotland) was shaped to coordinate the lead of the conflict, along these lines decreasing Essex's power as Lord General. Among the MPs named to this amazing panel was Oliver Cromwell. He was currently one of that little gathering of men who dominated: fifteen individuals from the Commons, seven Lords and four Scots. He was rising extremely quick indeed.

As yet, obviously, the new Eastern Association structure existed distinctly on paper and, as Cromwell composed, 'paper pays not, if not executed'. In the following not many months the unequivocal job was Manchester's, as he attempted to transform the statute of 20 January into the truth of Association depository and supply offices based at Cambridge. Since this implied upsetting the past connection between the Cambridge advisory group and the neighborhood specialists, it was normally despised by the last option. Manchester's representatives every now and again needed to manage bleak and uncooperative men, and it took all the Earl's solidness, impact and consideration to convince them to acknowledge this new and progressive situation. He could comprehend, and somewhat identify, with their disquiet about the manner in which neighborhood power structures were being invaded by energetic men of generally low societal position. In this manner, as Clarendon composed, he was 'never at fault for any inconsiderateness towards those he was obliged to persecute'. He superseded neighborhood interests since he saw no alternate method of raising a powerful armed force, yet his graciousness just as his own social standing pretty much made this mistreatment endurable. Presumably no one else had the combination of birth and character expected to bring it through. It was this managerial work which made the financial and strategic spine of the military which won Marston Moor and which, at last, filled in as an example of association for the New Model Army. It has been said that 'the Civil War was won by advisory groups'. This is exaggerating the situation, however the directors did basically guarantee that the Parliamentary leaders in the field were not in a tough spot when they confronted their Royalist partners. What happened then was up to the soldiers.

Meanwhile, obviously, the conflict proceeded. Cromwell took a functioning part in the skirmishing and maneuvering for position which happened in the disputable land between Oxford, the Royalists' capital, and Cambridge, the capital of the Eastern Association. Albeit military history specialists have would in general bind their consideration regarding the significant fights and attacks, these occasions truth be told shaped just a glimpse of something larger of common conflict. It was not such a lot of a solitary full-scale struggle as a progression of clumsy guerilla activities — experiences, encounters, ambushes and attacks — a sporadic example of limited canine battles. At this essential level military exercises had as much course as the inconsistent development of ducks on a lake. In one scene of this sort Cromwell drove 1500 men on a dairy cattle stirring endeavor which drove off a Royalist crowd from right under the noses of the Oxford garrison.

But it was in the north, because of the happening to the Scots, that the conflict was bubbling up to an emergency. The Earl of Newcastle had been caught in York by the Fairfaxes and the Scottish General Alexander Leslie, Earl of Leven, an intense elderly person with more experience of the hard trudge of crusading than the remainder of the administrators set up. However even their joined armed force, 20,000 in number, was not huge enough to finish the barricade of York. They kept in touch with the Eastern Association and first Cromwell with the mounted force, then, at that point, Manchester with the foot, came to help them. By early June 1644 York was cut off from the outside world.

King Charles couldn't realistically stand to lose York so he sent Rupert north with orders to ease the city and beat the agitators' militaries. On 30 June the Parliamentary commanders discovered that Rupert was a simple eighteen miles away at Knaresborough. Not set in stone at any expense, even that of raising the attack, to keep Rupert from adding Newcastle's powers to his own, they walked out to Long Marston, realizing that from that point they could order every one of the ways to deal with York from Knaresborough. Behind them the city post cheerfully ravaged the besiegers' lines, finding 4000 new combines of boots as well as cannons and ammo. More awful still, the associated commanders had gravely thought little of Prince Rupert. In an astounding day's walk of 22 miles he accepting his soldiers the extent that Thornton Bridge over the Swale and afterward south again to York. The city was assuaged; Newcastle and Rupert worked together. By sheer speed of thought and activity Rupert had accomplished the clearly impossible.

What was he going to do straightaway? Naturally disrupted by this development, the partnered commanders expected that he may strike south once more. Manchester, obviously, was worried for the security of his now unprotected Eastern Association. The Earl of Essex had left the Home Counties and was disappearing on a totally pointless pursuit in the south west. Who could determine what Rupert probably won't do if he somehow managed to combine efforts with the King's military in the Midlands? There lingered by and by the phantom of the Cavaliers walking on London. Thus, right on time next morning, 2 July, the unified powers started to move away toward Tadcaster to impede the courses toward the south. By and by they had neglected to divine Rupert's expectations, to see what was going 'on the opposite side of the slope'. Rupert's guidelines were to beat the renegade armed forces and still up in the air to carry them to fight. Prior to heading to sleep the earlier night he had made an impression on Newcastle requesting him to have his infantry prepared to walk by four AM. Rupert expected to see these men on Marston Moor by 9 a.m. what's more had they been there he would have had the option to assault while the partners were in miserable chaos, strung out for eight miles along the paths to Tadcaster. However, for an assortment of reasons — including Rupert's absence of politeness in his dealings with Newcastle — the infantry were not in position until four PM. As the hours passed Rupert saw his best possibilities of triumph get away. Frantically disappointing for him, it was likewise a nerve-wracking day for the cavalry in the united back watch, among them Sir Thomas Fairfax and Cromwell. As they sat tight for the principle body of their own military to return, they needed to watch out for Rupert, contemplating constantly whether or not he would choose to assault before Newcastle's foot came up.

By four o'clock the two armed forces were drawn up in fight position and just a fourth of a mile separated. The soldiers on the Royalist side numbered 18,000; on the partnered side something like 22,000. According to the perspective of numbers alone it was the greatest fight at any point battled on British soil. Rupert put his own pony under Lord Byron on the right where he realized it would meet Cromwell's. For albeit this moderately aged MP didn't have anything somewhat drawing nearer the youthful sovereign's standing as a fighter — and to be sure had never really merited it — his series of fruitful mounted force activities had fascinated Rupert. 'Is Cromwell there?' he asked enthusiastically. In the middle the two sides had, as was standard, put the majority of their infantry, with more rangers behind them.

Then came a respite, considerably more nerve-wracking than the former long stretches of readiness. The two sides enjoyed a few benefits which they were hesitant to forego by progressing. The unified armed forces were on a slight ascent while the Royalist position was ensured by a long trench and fence. On the Parliamentary side the officers recited songs; it assisted with facilitating the strain of pausing. At seven Rupert concluded that it was past the point of no return in the day for a significant commitment. 'We will charge them tomorrow first thing', he told Newcastle, and afterward resigned to eat his dinner in harmony. After the long, warm summer's day a tempest started to develop. At 7.30 it broke, and, as it broke, the entire united line pushed ahead. Without precedent for this mission the drive had been grabbed from Prince Rupert's grip. Cromwell's cavalry immediately improved of the Royalist forefront, seriously took care of by Lord Byron, however were then themselves checked by the appearance of Rupert, hungry for the fight to come and carrying with him a portion of his hold and his own lifeguard. Strangely Cromwell himself had little impact in this hotly anticipated conflict between his rangers and Rupert's. Very almost immediately he had experienced a blade twisted in the neck and he needed to pull out to have it dressed. In his nonappearance the Scotsman, David Leslie, assumed responsibility and after a long, hard battle put the Royalists to flight. Rupert it was subsequently said, got away exclusively by stowing away in a beanfield. It was now that the discipline which Cromwell had imparted into his mounted force was indispensable. They checked, re-shaped and, Cromwell with them again, searched about for new work to do.

Quickly to their right things were working out positively. Manchester's foot, on the left of the associated focus, was squeezing consistently forward. Be that as it may, past them all appeared to be lost. Sir Thomas Fairfax had gotten through the positions of Lord Goring's mounted force just to observe himself to be distant from everyone else. Behind him he could see a few units of Goring's pony seeking after the remainder of the unified traditional over the forehead of Marston Hill, dispersing onlookers as they went. Different units were dispatching many charges against the Scots on the right flank of the unified infantry. In the middle, Newcastle's foot, known as the Whitecoats or the Lambs inferable from their coats of undyed woolen fabric, had put Lord Fairfax's infantry to flight. Both Fairfax himself and the senior commandant, the Earl of Leven, were cleared along in the tide of fugutives.

at the war zone 'the fire, smoke and disarray of that day' caused a situation of absolute disorder. The greater part of the leaders on the two sides had disappeared and, concerning the wanderers, he composed, they were 'so many, so short of breath, so astounded, so loaded with fears, that I ought not have taken them for men, however by their movement, which actually served them very well'.

Then, through the tumult, an example gradually became noticeable. Sir Thomas Fairfax took from his cap the white band which recognized him as an individual from the unified armed force. Having disposed of his field sign he had the option to go unnoticed through the Royalist lines until he arrived at the space where Cromwell's rangers was re-framing. It was currently certain that Cromwell would need to challenge Goring's cavalry and that everything would rely on the result of this conflict. Cromwell and David Leslie drove their regiments around behind the fight lines. They viewed as a battered square of Scottish infantry still tenaciously opposing Goring's invasion. Until Cromwell showed up on the scene the Royalist cavalry more likely than not accepted that triumph was at that point theirs. They were no counterpart for a charge conveyed from so startling a course. They broke and escaped, leaving Cromwell possessing the field. All that presently remained was to butcher the Lambs. Newcastle's Whitecoats were encircled and miserably dwarfed. Be that as it may, despite the fact that they were offered quarter they denied it. The individuals who had been generally hesitant to go to the field were, eventually, the most hesitant to leave it. Just thirty of them made due. The rest kicked the bucket where they stood and battled. To one onlooker it appeared to be like their white coats, shining in the twilight, had been brought to fill in as their twisting sheets.

After the fight Cromwell composed 'Genuinely England and the Church of God hath had an extraordinary blessing from the Lord, in this incredible triumph given unto us, for example, the like never was since this conflict started … God made them as stubble to our blades … Give greatness, all the wonder, to God.' But Rupert had different thoughts; in his view the credit had a place with Cromwell. From now into the foreseeable future he was to call him 'Ironsides'.

6. New Model Army

MARSTON MOOR opened up the possibility of complete triumph over the King. To some it was a horrifying possibility. Beforehand the more safe pioneers on the associated side had accepted they were battling to save Parliament. Yet, since this had been accomplished for what reason did the Committee of Both Kingdoms encourage them to proceed with the conflict as opposed to looking for an arranged harmony with Charles? Among the stressed conservatives was Cromwell's own boss, the Earl of Manchester. 'Assuming that we beat the King multiple times,' he said, 'he would be King still and his family down the line, and we subjects still.' Cromwell's answer is a proportion of the hole which opened up between them throughout the mid year and harvest time of 1644. 'My ruler, assuming this be all in all, for what reason did we wage war from the get go? This is against battling ever henceforth. Assuming this is the case, let us bury the hatchet, be it never so base.' If every one of the commandants had been just not really settled as Cromwell the conflict would likely have been over by that harvest time. Be that as it may, at this point not certain what he was battling for, Manchester liked to sit idle — aside from maybe shield the un-compromised lines of the Eastern Association. Triumph, he accepted, could just prompt further disarray and disorder; it would bring conflict, not harmony. The proof for this conviction lay not far off, in the fights what separated the officials of his own military. On one side were the Independents driven by Cromwell; on the other the Presbyterians, driven by a Scottish official, Major-General Lawrence Crawford. In August 1644, while they rested at Lincoln, Cromwell attempted to cleanse the multitude of his rivals. A few Presbyterian officials were cashiered and Crawford himself just barely got away — Manchester needed to vow to seek after a more dynamic military strategy to save his major-general. This assault on individual Parliamentarians whose strict sentiments varied from his own was another takeoff for Cromwell. Already he had been remarkably lenient, utilizing the two Presbyterians and Independents inasmuch as they were able warriors. Without a doubt in a well known letter written in March 1644 he had guarded this arrangement to in all honesty Lawrence Crawford. 'Sir, the State, in picking men to serve them, fails to acknowledge their perspectives, assuming they be willing loyally to serve them, that fulfills … Take notice of being sharp, or excessively effectively honed by others, against those to whom you can protest little however that they square not with you in each assessment concerning matters of religion.' In this Manchester and Cromwell had been at one. The two of them needed 'authentic' officials. Warriors like the French colonel, Mazères, who required his ladies, drink, cards and dice were cashiered. Be that as it may, in picking the 'genuine' they didn't look too carefully at partisan contrasts. Why then in the late spring of 1644 did Cromwell change his mind?

The central explanation is that he was headed to it by the prejudiced mentality of the actual Presbyterians. It was they who started the cashiering. In addition, because of his colleague with the Scots at the attack of York, Cromwell turned out to be especially frightened by their inflexible demand that the English Church ought to be revamped along the lines they set down. At Marston Moor God had offered a hint. He, Cromwell, had tracked down favor in seeing the Lord. 'We never charged yet we directed the foe.' With added trust in the honorableness of his motivation Cromwell was ready to meet bigotry with narrow mindedness and to defeat the adversary inside his own camp. Gotten between the groups and excessively gentle tempered to have the option to force harmony upon them, Manchester became exhausted of a battle which appeared to be progressively inconsequential. Openings were lost. The increases made at Marston Moor discarded. In the far south west the Earl of Essex permitted himself to be moved into a corner at Lostwithiel. Cromwell noticed these occasions with developing restlessness. On 5 September 1644 he kept in touch with his brother by marriage, Colonel Walton:

We do with distress of heart hate the dismal state of our military in the West, and of issues there. That business hath our hearts with it, and genuinely had we wings, we would fly there. So soon as ever my Lord and the foot let me free, there will be no need in me to hurry what I can to that help ... we have some among us much delayed in real life ... Pardon me that I am in this manner irksome. I compose however sometimes; it gives me a little reassure to pour I, amidst slanders, into the chest of a friend.

But 'my Lord' didn't release him. Rather he said that 'assuming any ought to convince him to go toward the west he would hang him'. At last, when it was past the point where it is possible to save Essex's military, Manchester progressed, however just to the extent Reading, where he stayed for quite some time, disregarding both the directions of the Committee of Both Kingdoms and the critical solicitations for help sent by Sir William Waller who was pulling out eastwards in face of the prevalent Royal armed force. Not until 21 October did each of the three Parliamentary authorities, Essex, Waller and Manchester rendezvous at Basingstoke; their joint powers totalled nearly 18,000 men.

On 26 October Charles was brought to cove at Newbury. In spite of the fact that his military was feeling great after their victory at Lostwithiel, the best triumph of the conflict, it numbered just 10,000. The Parliamentary powers were obviously in a beneficial position, yet they were grieved by jealousies among the pioneers and consequently the general order was given, not to a solitary general, but rather to a Council of War from which Essex, attributable to ailment, was missing during the essential weeks. Charles involved a solid cautious position and a clear front facing attack was not feasible. It was chosen to send a large portion of the military, under Waller and Cromwell, on a long diversion, quite a bit of it around evening time, which would permit them to take the Royalists in the back. At the point when Manchester heard their firearms he was to dispatch a synchronous assault on the King's bleeding edge. Albeit the Royalists noticed Waller's surrounding walk and arranged a warm gathering, they were beaten back by the furiousness of the surge. Charles sent soldiers to mitigate the strain — and he could do as such without any potential repercussions since Manchester had not assaulted. In spite of the supplications of his officials he wouldn't move until over an hour after the sign had been given. By then it was past the point of no return. After a short time the sun set. Under front of obscurity the King removed his entire armed force and afterward pulled out to his very much braced winter quarters at Oxford while the Parliamentary powers rested. At the point when the King's getaway was found Waller and Cromwell were enraged. They requested a quick pursuit, yet Manchester would have none of it. On the Parliamentary side the following not many days were loaded up with sharp and unbeneficial questions. Subsequently on 9 November the King had the option to ease Donnington Castle, salvage the big guns train which he had been driven out behind during his hurried night retreat, and take it back in win to Oxford — this right under the noses of three Parliamentary militaries which, attributable to the lack of arrangements, were quartered excessively far separated to allow a quick grouping of forces.

The public clamor and interest for an examination which followed the help of Donnington Castle made it hard to hide the divisions which had portrayed the Council of War in late October and early November. The Earl of Essex, in the desire for reestablishing his own discolored notoriety, exploited his upheld nonappearance from the Council to assault its individuals in general, and afterward every one of them, in legitimizing his own behavior, was normally attracted to condemn the others. Waller and Cromwell were joined in censuring Manchester. On 25 November they conveyed their squabble into the House of Commons, with Cromwell openly blaming his own administrator for 'proceeded with backwardness to all activity'. In his answer Manchester demanded the aggregate liability of the Council of War however at that point, since it was hard

to assault Cromwell's tactical record, he focused on political and strict issues. Cromwell, he affirmed, detested their Scottish partners and was gone against on a basic level to a House of Lords; he planned to make a multitude of Independents, a military which could fill in as an instrument for extremist political activity. By raising the ghost of social disturbance Manchester had skilfully tested Cromwell's most weak flank. There was an inescapable dread that, as Essex expressed it, 'Our family will say that to convey them from the burden of the King we have exposed them to that of the commoners'. Of course, at whatever point King Charles felt discouraged he could perk himself up by pondering the divisions inside his foes' camp.

The peak to the fight was relied upon to come on 9 December when the Commons' advisory group set up to consider the charges against Manchester was because of report to the House. However, following the report was perused, Cromwell rose to make a speech.

It is currently an opportunity to talk, or always hold the tongue. The significant event presently is no not exactly to save a Nation out of a dying, nay practically biting the dust, condition, which the long continuation of this War hath currently brought it into ... For what do many say that were companions toward the start of the Parliament? Indeed, even this, that the individuals from the two Houses have extraordinary places and orders, and the sword into their hands; and ... will ceaselessly proceed with themselves in loftiness, and not grant the conflict expediently to end ... This that I talk here to our own countenances, is nevertheless what others do articulate abroad behind our backs ... If I might talk my soul without reflection on any, I do consider in case the Army be not placed into another technique, and the War all the more energetically indicted, the People can bear the conflict no more, and will uphold you to a shocking peace.

But this I would prescribe to your judiciousness, not to demand any grievance or oversight of any president upon any event at all; for as I should recognize myself at real fault for oversights, so I realize that they can seldom be stayed away from in military matters. In this manner postponing a severe investigation into the reason for these things, let us put forth a concentrated effort to the cure ... And I trust we have such obvious English hearts ... as no individuals from either House will second thought to deny themselves ... for the public good.

The discourse was a masterstroke. Instead of the quarrel against Manchester, Cromwell offered compromise; instead of a climate of unpleasant and damaging analysis, he proposed useful change. Scarcely any Parliamentary discourses have had so sensational an effect. Inside an hour the

Commons, dexterously controlled by Sir Henry Vane, had decided in favor of the drafting of a Self-Denying Ordinance — a standard that no individual from either House should hold any office, military or common, while the conflict lasted.

As a further immediate aftereffect of Cromwell's discourse the New Model Army was made. So particularly far as its arms, gear and strategies were worried there was to be nothing surprising with regards to the New Model Army. The development was to have a military which would battle anyplace, unencumbered by nearby ties. This necessary a concentrated monetary association, in view of Westminster, rather than an arrangement of money run by neighborhood or territorial panels — like the Cambridge Committee of the Eastern Association — which could keep down supply when they imagined that their own nearby advantages were being dismissed. In this sense the New Model Army was essentially an augmentation of the cycle which had seen the production of the multitude of the Eastern Association. It didn't seem OK to expect a military financed out of local assets to do a public job. Without a doubt it was the endeavor to do this, notwithstanding the monetary emergency which unavoidably happened, which to some degree clarifies the Association's moderately helpless military record after Marston Moor. At the hour of the Newbury lobby Manchester was attempting to keep ten regiments of infantry and forty soldiers of pony on precisely a large portion of the aggregate which Fairfax was given to keep twelve regiments and sixty soldiers in 1645. Be that as it may, with the possibility of triumph the opportunity had arrived to work on a public rather than a provincial scale. It was Manchester's refusal to see it in these terms which drove Cromwell to break with him. What was required now was an official corps with the viewpoint of expert warriors, not MPs or landed blue-bloods with one eye on their voting public and bequests. Toward the start of the conflict Cromwell's political base in the Fens was an extraordinary resource; so too was the Earl of Manchester's social remaining in East Anglia. Cromwell had the option to acknowledge the new circumstance; Manchester proved unable, or would not.

On 15 February 1645 the House of Lords hesitantly acknowledged the plan for the New Model Army. Sir Thomas Fairfax, neither a MP nor a companion, was named Commander-in-Chief; however the post of Lieutenant-General of the cavalry was left empty. The Lords' resistance to the Self-Denying Ordinance was fiercer and more drawn out. After each of the a MP could leave his seat on the off chance that he wished to hold his military order; no such choice was available to a friend. In this way not until 3 April did the Ordinance become law. In February and March Cromwell was still allowed to answer an invitation to battle. Sir William Waller had been given a multitude of 6000 pony and dragoons along with orders to diminish the

overwhelmed posts of the West Country. On 27 February Cromwell was shipped off go along with him. By 8 March they had arrived at Andover where they caught a little party of Royalists under Lord Henry Percy. What happened then is best left in Waller's own words.

Having att that time a badly designed sickness, I wanted Collonell Cromwell to entertaine him with some mutual respect; who did subsequently tell me, that among those whom we tooke with him (being around thirty), their was a young people of so faire a face, that he questioned of his condition; and to affirm himself willed him to sing; which he did with such a modesty that Cromwell scrupled not to say to Lord Piercy; that being a champion, he did shrewdly to be joined by Amazons; on which that Lord, in some disarray, did adknowledge that she was a maid; this a while later gave rise to scoffe att the King's party, as that they were free and wanton, and disapproved of their pleasure more than either their Country's administration, or their Maister's good.

n 10 March Waller discovered that a solitary Royalist regiment was quartered in and around Devizes. By walking during that time he overwhelmed them and by sending Cromwell ahead on a quick enclosing move he had the option to remove their retreat. Outsmarted and encircled, the Cavaliers set up just a symbolic obstruction, more than 3/4 of the regiment being taken prisoner. Before the month's over, regardless of steady badgering by Lord Goring's cavalry, Waller and Cromwell had connected with a formerly disengaged Parliamentary power under Major-General Holborn. This association accomplished, Waller then, at that point, turned north and walked to defy Goring, who pulled out to Bruton. After a fortnight of uncertain skirmishing the position had barely changed, however the two sides had figured out how to regard different's capacities. 'Honorable Lord,' composed Waller to Goring, 'God's approval be on your heart, you are the jolliest neighbor I have at any point met with.' In mid-April Cromwell and

Waller got back to London to set out their payments under the particulars of the Self-Denying Ordinance. It had been a troublesome mission. With its unpredictable interwoven of little fields the West was not mounted force country. As Waller composed, 'each field was just about as great as a stronghold and each path as undeniable as a pass'. However he had been given neither infantry nor cash to pay his mounted force and dragoons. In these conditions Waller did well to remove his and Holborn's soldiers securely. Be that as it may, for the antiquarian of Cromwell the main interest of this mission lies in the light it tosses on his person. Taking into account his issues with Lord Willoughby and

the Earl of Manchester it might have created the impression that Cromwell was an awkward or even a hazardous man to have as a subordinate official. This isn't the way, in later years — after a spell in one of Cromwell's penitentiaries — Waller was to recall and record his relationship with the future leader of England.

And here I can't however make reference to the miracle which I have oft times needed to see this hawk in his eirey: he att this time had never shown exceptional partes, nor do I feel that he did himself accept that he had them; for despite the fact that he was obtuse, he didn't bear himself with satisfaction or disdaine. As an official he was devoted, and did never debate my orders nor contend upon them. He did, to be sure, seeme to have incredible clever, and while he was careful of his own words, not advancing an excessive number of in case they ought to double-cross his considerations, he made others talk, until he had figuratively speaking filtered them, and known their deepest plans.

On his return from the West Country Cromwell was shipped off to war once more. Indeed, as per the last terms of the Self-Denying Ordinance as altered by the Lords, commissions didn't need to be surrendered until forty days from 3 April. A more significant Lords' alteration implied that there was currently nothing to stop an official, whenever he had set out his bonus, from being re-designated. Cromwell's prompt undertaking was to forestall King Charles moving his gunnery from Oxford to aid the help of Chester, which was being assaulted by Parliamentary soldiers. The Royalists intended to bring over an Irish armed force and to do this they needed to clutch Chester. Cromwell prevailed with regards to driving off the vast majority of the draft ponies in the Oxford region and constrained the King to amend his arrangements. All things considered the Royalists stayed feeling sure, and insight reports going to the Committee of Both Kingdoms clarified that the conflict was going to enter another basic stage. In these conditions the Commons chose to expand Cromwell's bonus for another forty days.

Fairfax, in the interim, had been laboring all through April to lick the New Model Army into shape. On paper he was in charge of a multitude of 22,000 men: 6600 mounted force, 14,400 infantry and 1000 dragoons. Albeit the mounted force and dragoons were promptly impending, it demonstrated difficult to raise anything like this number of infantry without falling back on impressment, and surprisingly then there were reasonably grave questions about the nature of the soldiers. Sir Samuel Luke composed, 'I think these New Modelers manipulate all their batter with beer for I never see so many savored my life in so short a period'. But

concerning the cavalry there were no such questions. After Marston Moor Leslie had said of Cromwell's pony that 'Europe had no better troopers' and these were the ones who gave the core of the New Model. Without a doubt the commitment of the Eastern Association to the New Model Army was an impressive one. In spite of the fact that set up out of three armed forces, Essex's, Waller's and Manchester's, eleven out of the New Model's 24 regiments were directed by Eastern Association officers.

On 7 May Charles left Oxford. Cromwell, with a power of 7000 men, was told to keep watch on the King's developments and guarantee that he didn't progress into the eastern districts. At this stage the conflict was being coordinated by the Committee of Both Kingdoms by a sort of controller. Other than containing men as protective in their standpoint as Essex and Manchester, the Committee's guidelines were unavoidably founded on outdated data. Cromwell and Fairfax were both compelled to make long, fast and unbeneficial walks trying to stay aware of the Committee's befuddled and once in a while problematic orders.

Not until the Committee was stunned into a feeling of authenticity by the news that the King and Prince Rupert had caught and sacked Leicester on 1 June, did matters improve. Fairfax was allowed to utilize his own on-the-spot judgment in choosing what course to take. Energized by this Fairfax utilized his own judgment to ask upon Parliament the need for naming Cromwell to the still empty post of Lieutenant-General. In a letter dated 8 June he composed: 'The overall regard and love which he hath both with the officials and fighters of the entire armed force, his very own value and the capacity for the work, his incredible consideration, determination and fortitude, and reliability in the help you have as of now utilized him in, with the consistent presence and gift of God that has went with him make us view it as an obligation we owe you and the general population to make our suit.' Without trusting that Parliament will support his solicitation, Fairfax kept in touch with Cromwell — who meanwhile had been shipped off arrange the guards of Ely — educating him regarding the arrangement and requesting him to enlist in the principle armed force immediately. The time had come to carry the King to battle.

The catch of Leicester had done Charles nothing but bad. Not just had it stirred Parliament right into it, it had additionally truly drained his own military. Other than the setbacks of the attack, there had been a post to find. In addition the sack of Leicester created such an excess of goods that a large number of the King's officers essentially vanished to partake in their portion of the plunder in

harmony. (It was unequivocally in light of the fact that effective pillaging prompted a breakdown of discipline that Cromwell was such a huge amount against it.) Thus with just 8000 men left, Charles had chosen to stand by at Market Harborough until he was supported by the powers under the order of Lord Goring and Charles Gerrard. As quite a while in the past as 19 May a message had been shipped off Goring requesting him to join the primary Royalist armed force. Lamentably Goring, albeit a fine mounted force authority — he had as of late fall off well in two or three encounters with Cromwell — was envious of Rupert and hesitant to serve under him. He would come, he answered, when he had caught Taunton. However, rather than proceeding with the attack of Taunton he focused on becoming inebriated. His nonappearance was to be significant. By contrast Cromwell, leaving Ely the moment he accepted Fairfax's letter, joined his Commander-in-Chief at six o'clock on the morning of 13 June. His appearance was announced 'a strong yell of bliss' from the rangers quarters.

That very evening Colonel Ireton astonished a Royalist station while the officers were nonchalantly eating dinner and partaking in a round of quoits. The caution was given and King Charles called from his bed at eleven o'clock. Until this reality check he had no clue about that his adversaries were so close. Briskly he gathered a 12 PM committee of war. In these conditions retreat would be troublesome, withdrawal may transform into embarrassing flight. However Rupert, ordinarily so anxious for the fight to come, prompted retreat. They would, all things considered, be dwarfed just about two to one. In any case, Rupert's expert assessment was overruled — as it had been so regularly in the beyond couple of weeks. The King tuned in rather to the contentions of two squires, Digby and Ashburnham, whose fight with Rupert was both infamous and lamentable. They poured disdain on the New Model Army and encouraged the King to turn and battle. At two AM the Royalist fighters were energized and told to set themselves up for battle.

Shortly after dawn on 14 June Rupert drew up his military on an edge south of Market Harborough. Be that as it may, on riding forward to notice the demeanor of Fairfax's powers, Rupert was bewildered by seeing Cromwell's cavalry creating some distance from him. Were the Parliamentarians pulling out? Basically it was maybe an opportunity to assault before they were prepared. Rupert communicated something specific requesting the remainder of the King's military to follow him and rode on, searching for a decent fight ground. What had indeed happened was that Fairfax had as of now drawn his military up when Cromwell saw that the ground before them was waterlogged. This, he contended, would not suit

cavalry and it may cause Rupert to rule against fight all things considered. 'Let us, I entreat you, step back to there slope, which will urge the foe to charge us.' Fairfax concurred and requested his soldiers to fall back to the edge behind them, Naseby Ridge. It was this development which had gotten Rupert's attention. Coordinated by Rupert the Royalist armed force progressed in fight request until it arrived at Dust Hill. The Parliamentarians had not relied upon to see the foe so far toward the west and not wishing to be defeated or to have the smoke of fight blown once more at them — for the breeze that day was north westerly

— they excessively moved west along Naseby Ridge until their left flank laid on Sulby Hedges. The militaries confronted each other across an open spread known as Broad Moor. Cromwell was presently furiously and joyfully occupied. Men saw him chuckling joyously and Cromwell himself reviewed his state of mind of that day. 'I proved unable, riding alone with regards to my business, however grin out to God in acclaims, in confirmation of triumph.' He was right at home; he exhibited the mounted force on the two wings. Ireton would order on the left while Cromwell himself took the right. Then, at that point, he rushed back a large portion of a mile to track down the dragoons under Colonel John Okey. They were expected to line Sulby Hedges. In the nick of time. Rupert, actually wanting to get the restricting powers cockeyed, had joined the cavalry on the Royalist right and presently he drove them in a difficult charge against Ireton — precisely as Cromwell had expected. Overcoming the flintlock fire of Okey's dragoons, and regardless of being dwarfed three to two, Rupert's mounted force cleared all before them. In any case, indeed the successful Cavaliers demonstrated difficult to control. Just their ravaging senses stopped them when they arrived at Fairfax's things train a mile behind the fight lines. Here Rupert was finally ready to re-structure his groups and persuade them back into action.

In the middle, in the mean time, the great Royalist infantry had additionally progressed nicely. However drained and dwarfed, they had prevailed with regards to getting through the Parliamentarians' cutting edge. To Fairfax's right side, be that as it may, where Cromwell told it was an alternate story. Here too the Royalist rangers, under Langdale, was dwarfed — and for once in the fight numbers were made to tell. The Cavaliers were directed. Cromwell itemized four groups to annoy them until they were dispersed past all desire for revitalizing. These pursuit units passed near King Charles' hold and the King himself needed to lead a counterattack, however was kept from doing as such by his sidekicks who dreaded for his life. The save dashed off in confusion.

Cromwell actually had the primary body of his mounted force flawless and on the front line. He swung them round to charge the unprotected left flank of the gallant Royalist infantry. This was simply the definitive stroke and presently Fairfax rode with them. Empowered by this development, Okey's dragoons remounted and charged in on the right like they were rangers. The Royalist foot had been left abandoned in a miserable position and albeit one detachment battled to the last, the greater part of them reasonably set out their arms and requested quarter.

It was now that Rupert got back with his hesitant horsemen. It was past the point of no return. He rode over to where the King was attempting to revitalize a few remainders of Langdale's rangers. They were seen by Cromwell's interest groups, yet these had orders not to connect with until the foot had been raised in help. Very much focused as ever they watched peacefully as Rupert and the King battled to change their lines. So for the second time that day two armed forces were drawn up in fight cluster. Be that as it may, on the King's side there was no infantry, nor could his enduring mounted force be convinced to charge. Only one volley from Okey's dragoons was sufficient. The Royalists turned and escaped, while the King and Rupert pointlessly endeavored to make them stand. Just the last pursuit, nearly to the doors of Leicester, remained. In any case, even this was a completely all around focused activity. Cromwell's troopers were requested not to get off for loot on torment of death. By contrast an observer saw a portion of the Royalists stop in their flight and hazard passing, to get cash spilt on the ground. It was a last, regrettable representation of the essential contrast between the different sides. On the Parliamentary side were the men whom Cromwell had picked and prepared. Peers were in no question on this score. Clarendon wrote:

That distinction was noticed not long after the start of the conflict, in the discipline of the King's soldiers and of those which walked under the order of Cromwell (for it was uniquely under him, and had never been famous under

Essex and Waller), that however the King's soldiers won in the charge, and steered those they charged, they never energized themselves again all together, nor could be brought to make a second charge around the same time ... though Cromwell's soldiers, in case they won, or thought they were beaten and by and by directed, mobilized again and remained neat and tidy till they got new orders.

aseby was won by Cromwell's veterans rather than by the New Model Army all in all, and the triumph showed even the dubious House of Lords that, while the conflict was on, Cromwell was indispensable.

Even so there may have been an alternate result to the fight — or no fight by any means — in case Goring had submitted to his guidelines. Here lay the prompt meaning of the Parliamentary changes helped through the previous winter. By demanding the cessation of the debate between the officers and making a unified order, they had, by political means, drastically changed the tactical circumstance. In the other camp there was Charles, whose powerlessness to control the political scene had prompted the episode of battle in any case. Furthermore it was exactly this powerlessness which had now guaranteed that he would lose the conflict. He was unable to control the squabbles of his commanders and subjects: Rupert, Goring, Digby and Ashburnham. By 1645 his court 'resembled a container of crabs, where every part battled for endurance against the rest' — and in their battles lay the harmful malignant growth which was to be the passing of the King's cause.

By overlooking the tragic leftovers of Charles' powers and directing their concentration toward Goring's undefeated armed force, Fairfax and Cromwell showed great key sense. Gutting had still not figured out how to catch Taunton which was held for Parliament by Robert Blake (later Admiral Blake, yet right now a man quick becoming master in the craft of standing firm on indefensible situations). At the point when he knew about the quick development of the New Model Army — moving nearly at Rupert's speed — Goring chose to raise the attack. By the morning of 10 July he had taken up a solid protective situation on the temple of a slope at Langport. For Fairfax's military, coming from the Yeovil course, the main methodology was to passage the stream at the foot of the slope and afterward move by the precarious slant of a tight path. Yet, Goring's musketeers lined the supports on one or the other side of the path while two weapons covered the actual passage. First Fairfax raised his cannons to quiet these two. Then, at that point, he sent in 1500 musketeers to cross the stream and clear a portion of the fences. Following an hour of furious skirmishing this had been accomplished. The scene was presently set for the peak of the fight, one of the most astounding of all cavalry charges, and one which Goring had plainly decided to be impossible.

airfax needed the cavalry to energize a path somewhere in the range of four yards wide, while Cromwell composed, 'our pony could hardly pass two side by side'. At the top, trying them to rise up out of the path, Goring's rangers remained on pause. The occupation was given to five soldiers of pony, every one of them drawn from Cromwell's own regiment. The assault was going by two soldiers under Major Bethell. They ran through the portage and up the path. They played out, the words are Cromwell's, 'with the best courage possible; beat back two collections of the foe's pony, being Goring's own detachment; brake them at sword point'.

But the force of the charge conveyed them profound into the foe lines until they were encircled and about to start being overpowered by prevalent numbers. They were saved by the appearance of three additional soldiers drove by Major Desborough. Then, at that point, a few musketeers additionally arrived at the forehead of the slope. Gutting's men probably thought that it is difficult to trust the proof of their eyes. Cromwell's troopers were not simply all around focused; they likewise had mental fortitude and energy. This, as Cromwell composed, 'gave such an unforeseen dread to the foe's military that set them each of the a-running'.

ith the trip of Goring's soldiers from the envisioned security of Langport the Civil War was basically at an end. Those powers which were still passed on to the King were depicted by Clarendon as being 'horrible in loot and undaunted in fleeing'. In the following nine months Fairfax and Cromwell, now and again working together, now and then independently, took out the Royalist palaces and towns of the south west individually. The Earl of Leven's Scottish armed force overwhelmed the north. In September 1645 Rupert, fatigued of court interest and a conflict without trust, given up Bristol. He encouraged Charles to sue for harmony. Yet, the King would not yield. In his answer to Rupert he showed the sort of honorability he was to require by and by — on the scaffold.

f I had some other fight yet the safeguard of my religion, crown and companions, you had full justification for your recommendation. For I admit that, talking either as to simple fighter or legislator, I should say there is no likelihood except for of my ruin. However, as to Christian, I should let you know that God won't endure dissidents to flourish, or His motivation to be ousted; and whatever individual discipline it will satisfy Him to incur upon me should not make me repine, substantially less to give over this quarrel.

With a miserably little armed force he meandered erratically around the Welsh Marches and the Midlands, on one event running east to sack Huntingdon. It did nothing but bad, yet to see the disappointment of Cromwell's old neighborhood might have managed the cost of him a specific horrid fulfillment. Not until June 1646 did Oxford, the Royalist capital, give up to Cromwell. Yet, Charles was no longer there. On 27 April he had his hair style short, put on a bogus facial hair growth and got out of Oxford around evening time. After some more desolate wanderings — this time with just two sidekicks — the King rode into the camp of the Scottish armed force at Newark and surrendered himself. He had concluded that, war having bombed him, he would need to proceed with the battle by different means. From Cromwell too it was time again to go to politics.

7. Of Levellers and Kings

THE First Civil War had been won, however the triumph had settled nothing. There were not very many men who could imagine England without a ruler and keeping in mind that each proposed harmony settlement incorporated a spot for the King, Charles had the option to keep each such settlement from being accomplished. He just needed to keep his assent. Consequently Charles was presently inquisitively like the ruler in a round of chess; for all intents and purposes weak, yet without him it was difficult to win. There could be no arrangement until you chose to play an alternate game, a game with new guidelines and no ruler. However, it was not for this that men had battled the Civil War. They had simply wished to ensure that the old game would be played their direction. To this degree Charles was imperative — and he knew it. He haggled with all gatherings, not determined to arrive at a settlement, but rather trusting by this means to upset the Independent-Presbyterian-Scottish union which had won the conflict. It was likewise a technique for acquiring time while he searched about for unfamiliar guide.

ost definitely, things went particularly as indicated by plan. The Scots held him for quite some time until, exasperated by his refusal to acknowledge Presbyterianism for longer than a three-year time for testing, they gave him over to Parliament in January 1647 and acknowledged £400,000 to cover the costs of their missions in England. Charles was passed on to Holdenby House in Northamptonshire; his excursion there was like a victorious advancement. It started to look like Charles and the Presbyterians in Parliament may settle — and terms which were detestable to an Independent like Cromwell. Yet, what could he do about it? Battle another conflict? Now Cromwell became sick. From the finish of January until mid-March Cromwell disappeared from the records of the House of Commons. On 7 March he kept in touch with Fairfax. 'It hath satisfied God to raise me out of a perilous ailment ... I got in myself the sentence of death that I may figure out how to confide in him that raiseth from the dead, and have no trust in the tissue.' It is evident that Cromwell was truly sick, and plausible that apprehensive strain had a lot to do with it. In any event, when completely reestablished to wellbeing, his disquiet is apparent from the genuine thought he provided for an arrangement to lead a military to Germany to help the Protestant reason there. Rather it was the military which drove him back into governmental issues, and not in Germany but rather in England.

With the Civil War over, the military may have been disbanded, yet with a Scottish armed force still on English soil and an insubordination in Ireland, it was judged

savvier to keep it in being. In being, yet neglected. By March 1647 the infantry's compensation was eighteen weeks falling behind financially, and the rangers' 43 weeks. This was all at once of pointedly rising costs and joblessness, when to be poor and without a task was a troubling possibility. For Parliament to treat, in this unceremonious style, the ones who had taken a chance with their lives in Parliament's motivation, and who knew that they merited better, was the surest method for transforming the military into a favorable place of extremist discontent. Many warriors were drawn in by the somewhat fair and libertarian thoughts of the Levelers, driven by 'Genuine John' Lilburne. There were even a few Levelers who accepted that Irishmen were equivalent to Englishmen. It was in the present circumstance that Parliament proceeded with its arrangements for disbanding the military, in the end offering the troopers a derisory a month and a half's unpaid debts of pay. Their unconstrained response was to choose specialists for go about as shop stewards for the benefit of the majority and present their complaints. These specialists were called 'Agitators'.

This improvement frightened Cromwell and the one who was day by day turning into his nearest political consultant, his child in-law, Henry Ireton. Despite the fact that they didn't go the extent that the Presbyterian bunch who conveyed a Commons' goal pronouncing that these Agitators were foes of the State, they were worried about a potential breakdown of armed force discipline. Subsequently Cromwell's words and activities were awkwardly uncertain and he experienced harsh criticism from both left and right. To

Lilburne it appeared to be that Cromwell was being driven by the nose by rapacious night crawlers'; to Clarendon it appeared to be that Cromwell was creating mischief in the military while claiming to belittle it.

Cromwell conducted himself with that uncommon dissimulation (in which he was an extremely incredible expert) ... he, when all is said and done, was sent a few times to make the military; where after he had remained a few days he would return again to the House and whine intensely of the extraordinary permit that was got into the army

... And in these and so forth talks, when he spake of the country's starting to be associated with new difficulties, he would sob sharply, and seem the most distressed man in the world.

To King Charles' pleasure the split between the military and Parliament extended. A few Presbyterians incubated a plot to send the King to Scotland and afterward force Presbyterianism with the assistance of a Scottish armed force. On 2 June 1647 the military held an overall get together at Newmarket and set out to oppose Parliament on the off chance that it became important. On 3 June a lesser armed force official, Cornet Joyce, later depicted by Fairfax as an 'curve Agitator', went to Holdenby House and assumed responsibility for the King. Cromwell surely knew and approved

of this progression. It was likely taken to keep Charles from going to Scotland. However, on 4 June Joyce went one phase further. He chose to move Charles to Newmarket. 'What commission have you to get my individual?' the King asked Joyce. The Cornet investigated his shoulder to where his fighters were standing. 'Here is my bonus. It is behind me.' 'It is,' answered Charles, 'as reasonable a commission and also composed as I have seen a commission written in my life.' It all complimented the King's feeling of being indispensable.

Since the military had shown that it would act with or without Cromwell, Cromwell chose to go with the military. He also went to Newmarket. There Fairfax and he set up an Army Council comprising of the commanders and four delegates from each regiment (two officials and two average Agitators). In any case, the Army Council was expected to be a discussion for political and strict discussion, with military authority remaining solidly in the possession of Fairfax's Council of War, where Cromwell and Ireton, rather than Fairfax himself, were the predominant players. Gradually the military moved towards London. Much to Cromwell's alleviation the Commons started to take a more mollifying line, however at that point the Presbyterian city horde helped support occasions. Following exhibits on the side of the

King, they attacked the Commons on 26 July and held the Speaker down in his seat while a goal calling upon Charles to get back to London was passed. Throughout the previous few weeks Cromwell had been opposing Agitator strain for a walk on London — 'an alluring snare to poor hungry fighters', as he depicted it. Presently, notwithstanding, he responded quickly. On 6 August Cromwell rode into London at the top of his cavalry.

possessing both London and the King — who was presently moved to Hampton Court — the military unmistakably held the drive. In any case, how might it manage it? Since June Cromwell and Ireton had been haggling with the King, no doubt stirring up a lot of alert for the more extreme individuals from the military. Charles' comment, that he thought that it is extremely difficult to believe the military officials since not even one of them asked anything for themselves, is one exceptionally striking outline of the hole between the King and a man like Cromwell. The dealings failed miserably, however added to the overall climate of doubt and vulnerability. In October the Levelers printed a declaration entitled The Agreement of the People which might have sold upwards of 20,000 duplicates and which imagined the finish of the government. In the Army Council discussions of that harvest time the split between the officers and the Agitators became wider.

On 11 November Charles broke parole and got away from Hampton Court.

No one knew where he had gone for sure his arrangements were. Cromwell exploited the disarray to reimpose his power over the warriors. One regiment stood up to. Cromwell had its chiefs captured and took a stab at the spot. Three of them were sentenced to death, yet they were permitted to toss dice for their lives and just the failure was shot. After that the remainder of the military submitted quietly.

King Charles, in the mean time, had stopped at Carisbrooke Castle on the Isle of Wight. From here he kept on haggling merrily with every invested individual, eminently Parliament and the Scots. At long last, on 26 December 1647, he closed terms with the Scots. The text of the arrangement, including the intrusion of one more Scottish armed force, was enclosed by lead and covered in the nursery of Carisbrooke Castle. At Westminster men realized that some arrangement had been finished up and on 3 January 1648 the Commons casted a ballot to sever relations with the King. Cromwell partook in the discussion. As indicated by a Royalist account he 'stood up, and the sparkle worm shimmering in his snout, he started to spit fire; and as Satan cited Scripture against our Savior, so did he against his sovereign, and told the House: "It is composed, Thou shalt not experience a two-timer to rule".

Then, at that point, he laid his hand on the handle of his sword.'

But who was to rule? Two of Charles' children were in Parliament's grasp: one of them, maybe? Or on the other hand ought to there be a republic? Or on the other hand was Cromwell proposing to be a tyrant? It is likely that he most definitely didn't have a clue about the responses to any of these inquiries. 'I can tell you, sirs,' he expressed, 'what I would not have, however I can't what I would.' Once again we carve out him stamping opportunity, holding back to witness what might, what the Royalists and Scots would do. Holding up was difficult. As the weeks hauled by both the military and the organization turned out to be increasingly disliked, to a great extent inferable from exorbitant costs and weighty tax collection following the awful reap of 1647. Following five years of abusive vulnerability, the King was starting to seem as though an image of pre-war request and security. News from South Wales gave a genuinely necessary spike to action.

On 1 May 1648 Cromwell heard that one of Parliament's commanders had been killed in a Royalist ascending in Pembrokeshire. On 3 May he walked from Windsor, taking with him three regiments of foot and two of pony. The Second Civil War had started, and without precedent for his life Cromwell had an autonomous command.

Two officials in Wales, Colonel Poyer and Colonel Laugharne, had wouldn't disband their regiments when requested by Parliament to do as such, and they

furnished the Royalists with some genuine military spine. All things considered, when Cromwell arrived at the scene, the dissidents had as of now been crushed in the field by Colonel Horton and had withdrawn into three of the grand palaces of South Wales: Chepstow, Tenby and Pembroke. Chepstow and Tenby gave up decently soon however Pembroke, held by Poyer and Laugharne, was an alternate suggestion. Cromwell showed up there on 24 May, however without substantial attack mounted guns he could gain no ground by any stretch of the imagination, regardless of tales that the post was starving and mutinous. Indeed Colonel Poyer kept his soldiers in surprisingly great request, however at that point he was a wonderful man — 'a man of two manners consistently; toward the beginning of the day calm and contrite, in the evening plastered and loaded with plots'. However he had plotted calmly enough to ascend from humble starting points to become city hall leader of Pembroke. Ultimately, after a progression of mishaps, one of which unloaded his big guns in the mud of the Severn Estuary, Cromwell's attack train arrived at Pembroke on 4 July. After seven days Poyer surrendered the inconsistent battle. The heads of the Welsh rising were shipped off London and sentenced to death, yet just one sentence was completed. A youngster drew parts. For the others the parts read 'Life given by God'; Poyer's paper was blank.

While Cromwell was confined in South Wales occasions were moving quickly somewhere else. There were riots in London; the armada mutinied; Kent and Essex rose. This kept Fairfax occupied in the south east. A party of northern Royalists, driven by Sir Marmaduke Langdale, held onto Carlisle, Scarborough, Pontefract and Berwick. They were nailed somewhere around the couple of regiments at the removal of Major-General John Lambert, however assuming the guaranteed Scottish intrusion had emerged in May or June when Cromwell and Fairfax had their hands full in far off corners of the realm, who knows what may have occurred. As it was, inside hardships postponed and disappointed the Duke of Hamilton's endeavors to raise a military. Not until 8 July did he cross the line, and surprisingly then he just had around 9000 men, a large portion of them undeveloped and poorly focused infantrymen. Wherever the Scots went they looted fiercely. They had carried such countless ladies with them that it was broadly accepted that they had come to claim the north and settle there. They progressed gradually, mostly on the grounds that the climate was horrifying, however predominantly in light of the fact that Hamilton was worried to get together with Langdale and give time for fortifications from Scotland to come in. Lambert, besides, battled a skilful back monitor activity. Hamilton may have put forth a greater amount of an attempt to carry the dwarfed Lambert to fight, yet he was all too

aware of his own absence of involvement as a general and permitted himself to be treated with scorn by his second-in-order, the Earl of Callander.

As soon as Pembroke had given up, Cromwell sent a large portion of his mounted force on ahead to join Lambert and afterward walked north himself with 3000 foot and 1200 pony. His frustrated infantry were in a sorry state and this gave hopeful Royalists a few reason for trust. 'Noll Cromwell is fallen into a lowland at Monmouth where his men uprising for need of pay, and will not budge;

... Satan a foot will these holy people mix.' But indeed the holy people walked, in spite of the fact that Cromwell needed to take them on a diversion through the Midlands to get 3000 sets of shoes and stockings. It was normal that the Scots would attempt to mitigate Pontefract, so Cromwell set out toward Yorkshire. On 12 August he worked together with Lambert among Leeds and Knaresborough; even presently they had under 9000 men. In the mean time the Scots, after much delay, had chosen to remain west of the

Pennines and on that day were currently at Hornby in Lancashire. At this point Hamilton was in charge of in excess of 17,000 men, however Cromwell's own gauge of the adversary powers ran as high as 24,000.

Cromwell then, at that point, struck across the Pennines. Regardless of the distinction in numbers, he was sure of the nature of his soldiers, and planned to carry the Scots to fight. On 16 August, at Hodder Bridge close to Clitheroe, he held a gathering of war. Hamilton's military was moving toward Preston, and the inquiry was whether Cromwell should cross the Ribble and walk south, corresponding with Hamilton's course, all together then to remain between the Scots and London, or regardless of whether he ought to strikingly proceed with his toward the west development winding up toward the north of the Scots and remaining among them and their base. It was the last course, removing the Scottish armed force's retreat, which offered the best any expectation of absolute triumph, and Cromwell took it. That evening his military set up camp in the recreation center of Stonyhurst Hall. Sir Marmaduke Langdale's power, 3000 foot and 600 pony, was quartered only three miles away watching the flank of the Scottish armed force. Just now, and excessively late, did Cromwell's rivals acknowledge how close he was. Over the most recent couple of days their insight had been staggeringly terrible. Therefore Hamilton's military was unstable in a long queue between Preston Moor and Wigan, seventeen miles toward the south. Indeed, even on the morning of the fight (17 August) Hamilton appears to have been either deceived or stupid for he requested the fundamental body of his infantry to cross the Ribble and walk on towards Wigan, accepting that Langdale alone could hold off Cromwell's attack.

Very early that day Cromwell had started the last phase of his development on Preston. Langdale's position was a solid one. The ground before him was damp and separated by fences — it made difficult work for Cromwell's cavalry. The fundamental street into Preston from Stonyhurst was depicted by Cromwell as 'a path extremely profound and sick'. By four o'clock, after some furious skirmishing, Cromwell was prepared to dispatch his fundamental assault. He sent two regiments of pony to hack their direction down the mud-filled path in what was 'as grimy a spot as I at any point saw ponies remain in'. However, the brunt of the battling was borne by the infantry whose work it was to progress on the two sides of the path, clearing the supports as they went.

n Cromwell's words, they 'did it with mind blowing boldness and goal … regularly coming to push of pike and to close terminating, and continually making the foe draw back ... the adversary making, however he was as yet worsted, extremely hardened and solid opposition'. Langdale's soldiers hung on with practically no assistance from the remainder of the military for over four hours, until in the long run their line imploded and they fell once more into Preston in disorder.

Sweeping into the town Cromwell's men held onto the Ribble span 'after an extremely hot debate ... at push of pike'. This assault left Hamilton himself with a back gatekeeper of mounted force abandoned north of the Ribble and cut off from the remainder of his military. On his orders the majority of the rearguard made off toward the north, sought after by a portion of Cromwell's cavalry. Hamilton, not really settled to rejoin his military, and showing colossal individual boldness, he and his guardian beat off the assaults of two soldiers of Cromwell's pony, and afterward swam across the downpour enlarged stream. They tracked down their infantry, under the skilled order of Lieutenant-General Baillie — one of the legends of Marston Moor — drawn up on Church Brow Hill. As night fell Cromwell's development troops caught the extension over the Darwen and afterward, at the foot of the slope, Hamilton's caravan. To the joy of the fighters one of the trucks was found to contain the duke's gold plate.

During the night Hamilton's infantry slipped unobtrusively away, unseen by Cromwell's depleted troopers. The Scottish rangers under Middleton had at this point got a critical message requesting its review from Wigan. The arrangement was that the two pieces of the military — both still relatively new since at this point they had taken no part in the battling — should meet on the Preston—Wigan street. Their predominant numbers should then demonstrate in excess of a counterpart for Cromwell's fight tired soldiers. Lamentably there were two Preston—Wigan streets and keeping in mind that the infantry walked down one, the rangers came up

by the other. In the haziness they totally missed one another. Without a doubt it was presumably Middleton's landing in the Darwen which stirred Cromwell to the way that the Scottish infantry had gone. Middleton turned and followed upon the tracks of the infantry, however presently, obviously, he was annoyed right by a portion of Cromwell's rangers regiments. Hamilton challenged not stop. His soldiers went through Wigan and set off southwards on a subsequent night walk. Cromwell's men went through the evening of 18 August in a field close to Wigan 'being extremely filthy and exhausted, and having walked twelve miles of such ground as I never rode in for my entire life, the day being exceptionally wet'. The following day the pursuit proceeded in the soil of the way to Warrington. In the end the Scots established a point of no return close to Winwick. Depleted and wet, half-starved and mud-covered, their numbers had dwindled quickly under Cromwell's determined tension in the last 48 hours. Additionally their 12 PM departure from Preston had implied abandoning a large portion of their ammo. However they battled, as Cromwell composed, 'with incredible goal for a long time; our own and theirs coming to push of pike and extremely close charges, and constrained us to give ground; yet our men, by the gift of God, immediately recuperated it, and charging exceptionally home upon them, beat them from their standing, where we killed around 1,000 of them, and took (as we accept) around 2000 detainees'. Hamilton and the remaining parts of his cavalry made off, passing on Baillie to make what terms he could. Cromwell conceded them — there were currently just 2500 remaining — their lives as a trade-off for every one of their arms and hardware. At Warrington Cromwell rested, passing on others to chase down Hamilton. 'Genuinely we are so bothered and wrangled out around here, that we can't accomplish more than walk a simple speed after them.' 'Badgering and wrangled out' for sure. The Battle of Preston was no set piece fight except for a multi day running battle in Old Trafford climate following hard upon a long walk from Wales to Leeds and afterward back over the Pennines. However his troopers did all that Cromwell requested that they do. Considering, as their commandant brought up, 'that a portion of these that are here, since fourteen days before I walked from Windsor into Wales have not had any compensation', it was an amazing exhibition. This was the New Model Army at its best in a magnificently ad libbed crusade. It finished the Second Civil War as certainly as the Naseby

— Langport crusade had finished the First.

It simply stayed to pound the last nails into the final resting place of the Royalist cause. After his fighters had partaken in a couple of days' rest Cromwell moved north once more. Carlisle and Berwick were as yet in Scottish hands, yet Scotland itself

was in strife. Energized by Hamilton's loss, old adversaries of his, driven by Archibald Campbell, First Marquess of Argyll, were offering to assume control over the public authority. On 21 September Cromwell crossed the Tweed and, once in Scotland, immediately found a sense of peace with Argyll. He thought that it is not difficult to converse with a man who rose at five each day and asked until eight. As a trade-off for the quick reclamation of Berwick and Carlisle he offered Argyll the help of the English armed force in his inside war. Lambert was sent ahead with a cavalry power sufficiently able to overawe Edinburgh while Cromwell remained behind to get the acquiescence of Berwick on 30 September. This done Cromwell walked to join Lambert. On 4 October he was ritualistically invited into Edinburgh. He remained there three days, in length enough to guarantee that Argyll was solidly introduced in power, and afterward got back to England via Carlisle.

here was another tactical errand left: the decrease of Royalist-held Pontefract. Cromwell was in no rush. He remained in and around Pontefract all through the entire of November; when he left, the palace was as yet not taken. What Cromwell had needed was not Pontefract, but rather time and distance

— time to decide on the thing to do straightaway, distance to keep him out of the bedlam of occasions in London. As he composed on 25 November, 'We in this Northern Army were in a holding up pose, wanting to see what the Lord would lead us to In his dispatch revealing the triumph at Preston Cromwell had communicated the expectation that 'they that are unyielding and won't avoid disturbing the land may rapidly be obliterated with regards to the land'. In any case, what precisely did this mean? How ought to be managed Charles I, the one who had set out to dive the country into battle briefly time, in rebellion of God's judgment as vouchsafed in his previous losses? It was before long evident that Parliament would not annihilate the agitators. Should the military shoulder the weight? Cromwell didn't know. Yet, while he faltered others acted. At their head was his child in-law, Henry Ireton. On 20 November the military's Council of Officers introduced to the Commons a Remonstrance drafted by Ireton. It requested that 'that capital and great creator of our difficulties, the individual of the King ... might be rapidly dealt with for the injustice, blood, and wickedness he is at fault for'. The Commons shoved the Remonstrance to the side, so the military set out to shove the Commons to the aside, or if nothing else to cleanse the House of those MPs who might not consent to the King's preliminary. On 6 December Colonel Pride, a previous brewer's drayman, remained at the entry to the House, grasping a rundown of those MPs who were considered politically questionable. He captured 45 and dismissed 96 others. The enduring MPs proceeded to meet and became known as the Rump Parliament.

That very evening Cromwell, after a relaxed excursion south, shown up in London. He said that 'he had not been familiar with this plan; at this point, since it was done, he was happy of it'. It required an additional three weeks, nonetheless, before Ireton at last convinced Cromwell that Charles needed to pass on. While he lived England could enjoy no harmony. On 1 January 1649 the Rump passed a statute setting up a court to attempt the King.

Once his brain was made up Cromwell was typically powerful in real life and eager in discourse: 'We will remove his head with the Crown upon it.' When Charles was brought to Westminster Hall on 20 January and the charge against him was perused out, Lady Fairfax bounced up and yelled 'It's completely false … Oliver Cromwell is a trickster.' She was hustled out of the court and the preliminary ambled on to its front appointed end. On 30 January King Charles' head moved on the framework at Whitehall. It was an incredible signal. Lords had been killed previously, either in the fieriness of fight or, with conscious mystery, in obscurity corner of some palace jail. Yet, this was the initial time in European history that a lord had been freely executed by his subjects. A few observers commented upon Cromwell's disposition of thrill in nowadays. He realized that he had passed the place of no return.

England was currently a republic, controlled by the ninety-odd MPs of the Rump — the shadow of a Parliament — and by the Council of State, an advisory group designated by Parliament. Its first, transitory President was Oliver Cromwell. One of its secretaries was John Milton. On 6 February the Commons had casted a ballot to nullify the Lords. 'It was rarely instructed,' they contended, 'that the entire country ought to be abused to keep up with the desire and mob of a couple drones.'

ut despite the fact that England took its new conservative status strikingly unobtrusively, there was as yet the topic of Charles I's different grounds, Scotland and Ireland. The day after the fresh insight about the King's demise arrived at Edinburgh, Charles II was announced King — King of Great Britain, France and Ireland. It was realized that the youthful King was aiming to increase his expectation in Ireland and that Prince Rupert, presently turned ocean skipper, had showed up off the Irish coast with a little armada. In Ireland the Catholic renegades, under arms since the time 1641, had made a collusion with the Protestant Royalists under James Butler, Earl of Ormonde. Just Londonderry, Dundalk and Dublin itself actually held out for

Parliament. An ironical Royalist paper, The Man in the Moon, imagined the capable and lively administrator of the Dublin post, Colonel Jones, restlessly watching out to the ocean for a first look at the focusing light of Cromwell's nose going to his assistance.

Clearly provoke activity was essential and, for once, the English government was not altogether engrossed by homegrown issues. On 15 March, three days after he surrendered the Presidency of the Council, Cromwell was designated to take order in Ireland. He was to have a military comprising of eight regiments of foot, three of pony and 120 dragoons. On

17 April the administrations of a youngster were called upon to attract parcels to conclude which regiments ought to go to Ireland. As per one record, nonetheless, 'they drew parts over and over, until fortune concurred with their longings'. One of the foot regiments would not acknowledge the decision of the lottery and the men tossed down their arms. To some extent it was the lasting issue of unfulfilled obligations of pay; partially it was a Leveler-propelled feeling of frustrate with the new government. Where were the social and lawful changes what men had trusted would follow upon the passing of the King? 'They' had executed Charles, just to have his spot. In the expressions of a contemporary bulletin: 'It's anything but an open foe that subjugates them, not damme Cavaliers, nor inflexible desirous and sullen Presbyters, however strict and Godly companions, that have supplicated, proclaimed and battled together for opportunity with them, that with their blades have cut in divide the chains of different Tyrants, but then presently are turned into the best Tyrants'. Furthermore the best of these was Cromwell. Numerous Levelers found Cromwell's conviction that he was just taking care of God's important responsibilities especially hostile. 'You will scant address Cromwell about anything, yet he will lay his hand on his bosom, hoist his eyes, and call God to record. He will sob, wail and atone, even while he doth destroy you under the fifth rib.' The title of one of John Lilburne's leaflets places their mistake more or less: England's New Chains Discovered.

In the aggravations of spring 1649 we can maybe recognize the far off starting points of Women's Lib. On 23 April,

a huge number of ladies held up upon the House with a request of around 10,000 hands to it ... and an individual from the House coming out requesting what the matter was with the ladies, the Gentlewoman that was to introduce their Petition replied, they were accompanied a Petition; he told her that it was not really for ladies to appeal, that they may remain at home to wash their dishes; she replied, 'Sir, we have scant any dishes passed on us to wash, and

those we have we don't know to keep them'. Another part told her it was abnormal that ladies should request; she replied, 'Sir, that which is unusual if not accordingly unlawful, it was bizarre that you remove the King's head, yet I guess you will justifie it'.

The rebellions of early May, if less odd, were all the more quickly disturbing. At Salisbury two regiments wouldn't walk to Ireland until England's own freedoms were gotten. These men wore the Leveler's colour

— cean green — in their caps. Comparative in soul was the revolt driven by Captain Thompson at Banbury. To the Levelers it appeared to be that Cromwell, earlier a resistance chief and subsequently a decent 'Ocean Green Man' had demonstrated all around effortlessly defiled by the force of the blade. Cromwell's own demeanor was uncovered precisely enough in Lilburne's record of the Council of State's examination concerning his pamphleteering. In the wake of being questioned Lilburne left the room. Behind him he could hear Cromwell pounding the table and shouting: *I tell you, you have no alternate method for managing these men yet to break them or they will break you ... and baffle and make void all that work that, with so many years' industry, work, and torments, you have done, thus render you to all judicious men on the planet as the most terrible age of senseless, discouraged men in the earth to be broken and directed by such an abominable, disgusting age of men as they are ... I tell you once more, you are required to break them.*

n this soul Cromwell and Fairfax set out on 1 I May to break the mutineers.

Cromwell was sent on ahead with two regiments of rangers and he moved quicker than at some other time in his life. The evening of Sunday 13 May, having ridden all of 45 miles that day, he found the most difficult of the double-crossers at Burford. There was a short fight in the haziness however Cromwell enjoyed the benefit of shock and overpowering strength. In the blink of an eye at every one of the rebels were broken and directed. A few of them were killed. A couple got away, among them Captain Thompson. The rest, almost 400, were kept secured up Burford Church from Sunday night until Thursday. Then, at that point, they were delivered so they could watch the terminating crew manage three of the instigators. A fourth instigator, however sentenced to death, was reprieved without a second to spare when he uncovered that he had invested his energy in Burford Church composing a handout against insurrection. Thompson escaped across country and was ultimately caught in

a wood close to Wellingborough. However, he wouldn't give up. Twice he attempted to get through the cordon and was crashed once again into the wood. On the third endeavor he was shot dead. On the day that Thompson passed on Cromwell and Fairfax were ritualistically invited to Oxford to have the level of Doctor of Civil Law gave upon them by that most Royalist of universities.

8. The Lord of Hosts

ONCE the Levelers had been taken care of Cromwell was allowed to focus on his Irish campaign. Ireland had been the cemetery of numerous an overall's standing and not set in stone not to experience a similar destiny. Not until he was happy with the game plans for paying and provisioning the military would he leave. In case he succeeded where before administrators had bombed it was generally on the grounds that his officers were better taken care of, regardless of the way that he was working in a wide open squandered by numerous long stretches of war. When of his takeoff from London in July 1649 he had set up for more than £600,000 to be made accessible for the military in Ireland. He waited over the excursion to Milford Haven, hanging tight for a portion of the guaranteed money to find him. It isn't is to be expected that Ormonde said he dreaded Cromwell's cash more than Cromwell himself. On 13 August Cromwell set forth. As per his clergyman even before their boat left harbor he was 'as ocean debilitated as ever I saw a man in my life'. This separated he had a long list of motivations to feel bright, having right away before got news that Colonel Jones had broken out of Dublin, assaulted Ormonde's camp at Rathmines and won a devastating triumph. 'A shocking leniency,' composed Cromwell, 'so incredible and opportune that we resemble to them that imagined.' accordingly Ormonde couldn't place a military into the field against Cromwell, and the endeavor turned into a mission of attacks rather than one of battles.

On showing up in Dublin Cromwell delivered a discourse wherein he discussed 'carrying on the extraordinary neutralize the savage and murderous Irish … engendering the Gospel of Christ — and reestablishing that draining country to its previous bliss and serenity'. He had come to Ireland in light of the occasions of 1641, expecting to 'rebuff the most primitive slaughter that consistently the sun observed'. Anyway he didn't view all Catholics as being similarly liable, making a differentiation between the nobility whom he considered to be the creators of the resistance and the tenantry who were simply their hoodwinks. Since Catholics involved more than four-fifths of the all out populace this was maybe comparably well. In the light of this differentiation Cromwell put forth attempts to accommodate the Irish proletariat to the presence of his military. Pillaging was totally precluded; two fighters discovered taking hens were hanged. Ranchers were welcome to carry their produce to the military and were conceded assurance and installment in prepared cash. For this framework to work, obviously, the warriors must be paid consistently. All things being equal, the country economy of Ireland was not adequately evolved to have the option to help a multitude of 12,000 for long. The wide open was wild; there were a lot of wolves, yet too couple of individuals. As one seventeenth-century voyager put it, the Emerald Isle resembled 'a youthful vixen that hath the green disorder for need of possessing'. Militarily this implied that Cromwell's procedure was molded by his need to stay in contact with the armada on which he depended for supplies.

After Rathmines Ormonde had removed toward the north, thus it was northwards that Cromwell turned on leaving Dublin on 30 August. The main significant hindrance was the sustained town of Drogheda, thirty miles away at the mouth of the stream Boyne. The authority of the 2500 men of the Drogheda post was Sir Arthur Aston, an expert fighter who had seen administration in the mainland wars. Since, as Aston would like to think, the one 'who could take Drogheda could take damnation', he was certain that he could hold the town until the two boss foes of all blockading militaries — Ormonde called them Colonel Hunger and Major Sickness — constrained Cromwell to resign. In the new past Drogheda had demonstrated a difficult one to figure out, however for Cromwell taking it was crafted by a second. This was on the grounds that his careful arrangements had incorporated an astoundingly exceptional cannons train. Consequently Cromwell didn't need to settle down to the long bars so normal for fighting abroad. He would make a break in the dividers and afterward attempt to overwhelm the spot. One brief battle, but bleeding, cost him less lives than did the illness chaperon upon a tedious attack. Notwithstanding the use on attack big guns this strategy, inferable from the time saved, additionally cost less cash — a point which Cromwell knew would interest Parliament. After he had been eight months in Ireland he kept in touch with the Commons, 'Those towns that are to be diminished, particularly a couple of them, assuming we ought to continue by the guidelines of different states, would set you back more cash than this military hath had since we came over. I trust, through the gift of God, they will come less expensive to you.' An extra benefit moved by Cromwell was his order of the ocean — Prince Rupert's armada was barricaded in Kinsale Harbor by Admiral Blake. This allowed him to move his attack firearms to Drogheda by transport. By 9 September they were in position and he chose to begin the barrage next morning. Instantly at eight o'clock a message was shipped off Aston, expecting him to give up to forestall superfluous death toll. Aston declined. The firearms started to play.

y five o'clock the next evening (11 September) the divider had been

penetrated in two spots. Then, at that point, the raging gatherings were sent in. They were beaten back once owing, as Cromwell kept in touch with, 'the benefits of the spot and the fortitude God was satisfied to give the safeguards'. Yet, at the second endeavor they constrained their direction into the town. Now, obviously, sheer weight of numbers told in support of Cromwell. A portion of the post, including Aston, withdrew to a strongpoint known as Mill Mount. What happened then was subsequently recalled by Cromwell in serenity: 'Our men getting dependent upon them, were requested by me to put them all to the blade. Furthermore without a doubt, being in the fieriness of activity, I restricted them to save any that were in arms in the town, and I think, that evening they put to the sword around 2000 men.' Among them was Sir Arthur Aston, beat to no end with his own wooden leg. Others took shelter in the steeple of St Peter's Church and would not give up. Cromwell requested the spot to be exploded, and when this fizzled had the wooden seats heaped under the steeple and set land. Nearly fifty attempted to get away and were killed. The rest kicked the bucket as the blazing woods, rooftop and chimes came smashing down. As Cromwell saw in his dispatch to the Commons, 'One of them was heard to say amidst the flares: "God damme me, God jumble me I consume, I consume"'. His own misfortunes Cromwell assessed to be around 100, with a lot more injured. The entire scene was 'a noble judgment of God upon these savage miscreants', obviously it was identified with the future just as the past. It was implied as a notice to other people, explaining the results of their inability to give up and acknowledge quarter when it was proposed to them. The fact is made in a brief note kept in touch with the legislative leader of Dundalk on the day after the slaughter of Drogheda:

ir,

offered benevolence to the post of Drogheda, in sending the Governor a request before I endeavored its taking, which being declined brought their evil upon them.

f you, being cautioned accordingly, will give up your post to the utilization of the Parl of England, which by this I gather you to do, you may subsequently forestall radiation of blood. If, after rejecting this deal what you like not comes upon you, you will realize whom to fault. I rest,

Your worker,

Oliver Cromwell.

As well as being reasonable as far as military practicality, Cromwell's activity was authentic in however much it fell inside the structure of the

globally acknowledged laws of war. To be sure, in the event that a post denied quarter, the ones who had, accordingly, been constrained to chance their lives in an attack, reserved the privilege to sack the city and put every one of the occupants to the sword. As the renowned seventeenth-century law specialist Grotius, put it, 'the butcher of ladies and youngsters is permitted to have exemption, as understood in the law of war and the 137th Psalm — "Glad will he be that taketh and dasheth thy kids against the tempest"'. Drogheda was not sacked nor — with one exemption — was there any approach of killing the regular people inside its dividers, however some without a doubt more likely than not died in the grisly disarray. The exemption lay in the way that Catholic clerics and ministers were killed. Unmistakably Cromwell was bound to demand those privileges permitted him by the laws of war when Catholics were involved. The main spot in England which had been given anything like the Drogheda treatment during the Civil War was Basing House, the incredible chateau which was the focal point of Catholicism in the south.

ere we have one of the keys to understanding the standing which Cromwell 'appreciates' in Ireland. Drogheda should be taken a gander at in the light of military rationale and the laws of war, yet it likewise has a place in an air of dread and scorn — of Protestant against Catholic, English against Irish. It was this environment which had made the legend of the Irish slaughters of 1641; it was a similar climate which loaned the characteristics of amazing barbarity to the killing of the Drogheda post. Aside from proficient history specialists nobody in England today recalls the 1641 legends. Nobody has motivation to; after Cromwell the English were on the triumphant side. However, the Irish Catholics were the failures in the seventeenth century and were to stay the washouts for the following 300 years. It is in the minds of the persecuted that these accounts, whether or not precise, stay clear and significant. Accordingly for the Irish the name Drogheda has the sort of ring which the name Hiroshima has for those abused by the risks of atomic conflict. In the two cases, transient military benefit was purchased at gigantic mental cost.

From Drogheda Cromwell sent one separation to the help of Londonderry, while he and the remainder of the military — somewhere in the range of 9,000 men

— turned south. By 10 October they were digs in external Wexford and the attack weapons, postponed for seven days by storms adrift, were in position neglecting the town. Next morning the batteries started shooting and inside a couple of hours the legislative leader of Wexford, David Sinnott, consented to examine give up terms. Yet, during the dealings, one of Sinnott's agents, the skipper of Wexford

—

Castle, 'being genuinely treated', as Cromwell put it, 'yielded up the palace to us, upon the highest point of which our men no sooner showed up, however the foe stopped the dividers of the town, which our men seeing, ran fiercely upon the town with their stepping stools, and raged it ... our powers brake them, and afterward put all to the blade that came their direction'. In Cromwell's assessment he lost not in excess of twenty men, while almost 2000 Irish were killed. He had expected to give them reasonable terms, 'yet God would not have it so ... however in His honorable equity, brought an only judgment upon them'. The uncontrolled slaughter of Wexford, following close upon the controlled slaughter of Drogheda, broke Irish obstruction for some time. 'It isn't to be envisioned,' composed Ormonde, 'how incredible the fear is that these triumphs have struck into this individuals. They are stupified to the point that it is with extraordinary trouble that I can convince them to act anything like men.' Many of the ports of Southern Ireland, Cork among them, chosen to move their loyalty to Parliament without hanging tight for Cromwell's appearance. His aim was 'to follow Providence in indicting the adversary whiles the dread of God has arrived'. In view of this he laid attack to Waterford on 25 November.

But in the event that Providence was Cromwell's ally, the components surely were not. The downpour was unrelenting; the stockpile ships were held up by storms; many troopers fell wiped out — 'a significant piece of the military is fitter for an emergency clinic than the field; on the off chance that the adversary didn't have any acquaintance with it, I ought to have held it impolitic to have writ it'. Cromwell himself had been, as he put it, 'insane in my wellbeing'. Because of infection and the need to post recovered towns Cromwell's military was presently diminished to a successful battling power of 3000 men. The post of Waterford realized it obviously, and were not arranged to surrender.

On 2 December the besiegers pulled out, 'it being as awful a day as ever I walked in'. The time had come to go into winter quarters. Cromwell had driven his warriors hard, maybe excessively hard. Three weeks sooner he had brought up that the English had until recently never pursued a colder time of year battle in Ireland. However he knew this, he gave his fighters very little reprieve, brief period to recuperate their wellbeing. Cromwell was a man in a rush. He needed to 'hurry to the furthest limit of our work, as the worker doth to be very still'. He realized that his essence was needed in England and he wished to finish his work before he was formally educated regarding Parliament's desires. Additionally he didn't know for how long Parliament would acknowledge the substantial monetary requests forced by the Irish conflict. It had effectively cost about £700,000 and Cromwell's dispatches are loaded with demands for more cash. The crushed Irish wide open could

scarcely produce sufficient cash to pay for the posts. To keep the field armed forces in being English assets were key — among them, for instance, two entire shiploads of cheese.

On 29 January 1650 reinforced by the appearance of newcomers and new supplies from England, yet tormented by 'sore and stormy breeze and downpour', his military walked out of winter quarters.

Apart from the retreat from Waterford the undertaking had so far gone quite a well, however the area acquired had all been seaside since Cromwell had been hesitant to wander a long way from his stockpile ships. Presently the point was to drive inland to Tipperary and Ormonde's old HQ Kilkenny. The technique was to raise attack weapons and power many palaces to give up. Each palace acquired implied region lost for the foe and hence a further decrease in his assets in men and cash. It was the standard technique for archaic fighting, with weapons got to hurry the work. The powers went against to Cromwell, under the ostensible administration of Ormonde, were indeed in such political and strict disorder as to make it unimaginable for them to gather a military large enough to forestall this piecemeal victory of domain. Kilkenny itself fell toward the finish of March. However it was amusingly right now of triumph in Ireland that Cromwell endured what was likely the greatest interfered with of his entire military profession. Toward the finish of April, in what more likely than not appeared to be a minor wiping up activity, he drove his soldiers to the strengthened town of Clonmel where a post of 1200 under the order of Hugh O'Neill actually waited. Cromwell's firearms took care of their standard business of making a break in the town dividers, however rather than attempting to fix the break, O'Neill utilized stones and lumber to develop dividers on one or the other side of an entry driving back nearly eighty yards from the break. Toward the finish of the entry he burrowed a trench and set his firearms there. At the point when Cromwell requested a tempest the assaulting troops were permitted through the break unhindered, yet they then, at that point, wound up in a passing snare, enduring an onslaught from three sides, and kept there by the tension of their own men progressing behind them. The English misfortunes were weighty, however it is hard to give an exact figure since — maybe essentially — Cromwell didn't portray the Clonmel scene in one of his standard dispatches to Parliament. However in spite of the fact that he neglected to overwhelm Clonmel his unrivaled assets and cautious arrangements demonstrated adequate. O'Neill ran out of ammo and walked covertly out of the town around evening time. Next morning, 18 May, Clonmel's city hall leader surrendered.

By now it had become difficult to overlook the note of desperation in the

requests for Cromwell's re-visitation of England. His undertaking to Ireland had settled the destiny of that country. In spite of the fact that there was still some incomplete business it was, in military terms, of optional significance. There would be little brilliance in it, just — assuming that Clonmel was anything to pass by — irritation. So on 26 May Cromwell cruised away, leaving Henry Ireton in control. In November he had told the residents of Waterford that he had 'come into these parts, not to obliterate individuals and spots, however to save them, that men might live serenely and joyfully'. On the off chance that such at any point were his aims, he had fizzled, and the ones who proceeded with his arrangements bombed moreover. It has been assessed that in these years 33% of the complete Irish populace kicked the bucket because of war, plague and starvation. Irishmen would not fail to remember the nine months he spent in their midst.

In 1650, in any case, Englishmen completely endorsed Cromwell's fruitful disappointment in Ireland, and right from Bristol to London they gave him a saint's gladly received. Cromwell, obviously, gave all the credit to God. Parliament listened joyfully to a speech in recognition of Cromwell's accomplishment — and therefore needed to delay thought of an Act against ladies who painted their countenances, wore dark patches or improper dresses.

At about a similar time, a man who rather enjoyed shameless dresses, Charles II, at last decided that assuming he wished to sit on his lofty position he would need to look for the assistance of a Scottish Presbyterian armed force. This choice had for quite some time been normal by the English Parliament and it was predominantly to plan for this possibility that Cromwell had been called back. Not that Cromwell would essentially be Commander-in-Chief against the Scots. Fairfax, all things considered, was as yet the senior official. However, Fairfax had become progressively uncomfortable with the occasions of the most recent eighteen months and, not being a legislator by personality, his response was to pull out, passing on the stage to men like Cromwell. In June he declared that he would not lead an attack, and all endeavors to make him adjust his perspective — including those made by Cromwell

— were to no end. In a conversation which went on until quite a bit later

Fairfax stayed consistent. Cromwell contended that since Charles had joined the Scots they will undoubtedly attack soon. 'That there will be battle between us, I dread, is unavoidable. Your Excellency will before long decide if it will be smarter to have this conflict in the insides of another nation or of our own.' In his answer, Fairfax conceded that 'it is likely that there will be battle between us, however regardless of whether we should start this conflict and be the hostile part, or just stand

—

—

upon our protection is what I compunction'. More likely than not Fairfax was happy of a decent reason to go into retirement, while the legislators probably been mitigated that so troublesome a task was at this point not in the possession of a weak general. Not even Cromwell could move toward this errand with the ethical enthusiasm which he had brought to the Irish lobby. In long affirmations he disclosed to the Scots that he was attacking their country out of unadulterated warmth for them. In a letter kept in touch with Ireton he summed up the substance of these presentations. 'We made extraordinary callings of adoration, realizing we were to manage numerous who were Godly; the Lord helped us to sweet words, and in earnestness to mean them. We were dismissed over and over, yet still we implored them to accept that we cherished them as our own spirits.' The issue was summarized in the people of the two administrators. The Scottish general was David Leslie — he and Cromwell had battled next to each other in the left wing of the cavalry at Marston Moor; to be sure it might well have been Leslie who made all the difference when Prince Rupert appeared to be conveying all before him.

On 22 July 1650, with a multitude of 16,000 men, half infantry, half rangers, Cromwell crossed the line. In the entire country among Berwick and Edinburgh he tracked down little food and no men under sixty; both had been collected by the Scots and removed to Edinburgh to support their own military. Cromwell's officers were looked by young men who expected to lose their right hands and ladies who expected to have their bosoms cut off — for such were the monstrosity stories to which the conduct of the English armed force in Ireland had given ascent, and which absolutely had an all the more remarkable impact on the minds of terrified individuals than Cromwell's over-long protestations of selfless love. Again Cromwell had to depend on supply ships to keep his military in being, yet his arrangements were, of course, fastidious, deserving of King Edward I, the Hammer of the Scots. So to be sure were Leslie's. He had set up a solid guarded line from Holyrood to Leith and didn't, at this point, plan to come out from behind it to face a pitched conflict. As Cromwell composed, 'I accept they would prefer to entice us to endeavor them in their speed, inside which they are dug in; or probably trusting we will famish for need of arrangements; which is probably going to be, assuming we be not ideal and completely provided'. Leslie was more right than wrong to be wary. Albeit the powers available to him were better in numbers than Cromwell's, the nature of a considerable lot of them was dubious. In addition while Cromwell was obviously ace in his own home, Leslie was continually aggravated by the manner in which an advisory group of Presbyterian

government officials meddled with his treatment of the military. On one such event, Leslie and his Lieutenant-General 'took their fit and disappeared in a passion'.

Nonetheless the initial five weeks of the mission worked out positively for Leslie. There appeared to be no chance wherein Cromwell could compel the Scots to battle on ground which they knew obviously better than he and where — as one of his officials clarified — the passes were 'so many thus incredible that when we go on the one side they go over on the other'. As Cromwell sneaked forward and backward like a monster of prey looking for where he could jump upon his foe, yet never setting out to leave his stockpile ports — Musselburgh and Dunbar — a long ways behind, his troopers experienced their openness to the Scottish summer and from the provocations of adversary skirmishing parties. Two sections from one of Cromwell's dispatches uncover what these weeks resembled for the English.

e lay still all the said day; which ended up being so sore a constantly of downpour as I have only here and there seen, and extraordinarily to our inconvenience, the foe having enough to cover them, and we nothing at all impressive. Our officers stood this trouble with incredible fortitude and goal, trusting they should quickly come to battle. Toward the beginning of the day, the ground being extremely wet, our arrangements scant, we set out to step back to our quarters at Musselburgh, there to invigorate and revictual.

The adversary, when we drew off, fell upon our back and put them into some little issue ... We came to Musselburgh that evening, so drained and wearied for need of rest, thus grimy by reason of the wetness of the climate, that we expected the foe would make an infall upon us, which appropriately they did, somewhere in the range of three and four of the clock in the morning.

n these conditions it isn't is business as usual that an English official ought to have depicted Cromwell's men, as they lay digs in at Dunbar on 1

September, as 'a poor, broken, eager, debilitate armed force'. In numbers they were currently down to 11,000. It was the ideal opportunity for Leslie to head toward the assault. Following day 23,000 Scots involved Doon Hill, almost two miles away and controlling the street out of Dunbar. This, in a letter to Sir Arthur Haselrig, is the means by which Cromwell evaluated his position.

To the Honorable Sir Arthur Haselrig at Newcastle or somewhere else.

Scurry, haste,

Dear Sir,

e are upon a commitment truly challenging. The foe hath obstructed our direction [to Berwick] at the Pass through which we can't get without nearly a

wonder. He lieth so upon the slopes that we realize not how to come that way without incredible trouble; and our lying here day by day consumeth our men, who fall debilitated past creative mind ... Do you get together what drives you can ... ship off companions in the south to assist with additional. I would not disclose it, in case peril should accumulate accordingly.

In spite of this Cromwell composed, in a similar letter, that 'our spirits are agreeable (commended be the Lord)'. Finally it looked like he planned to get what he had come for — a fight — and assuming the Scots planned to assault they would need to descend from the strategic position. Around four PM Cromwell and his officials, chief among them Major-General Lambert and Colonel Monck, noticed — with the guide of their point of view glasses — a slight development in the Scottish camp. They were coming down to take up a position prepared to assault on the morrow. 'God is conveying them into our hands,' said Cromwell, 'they are coming down to us.' But in the Scottish camp the pioneers were similarly sure, without a doubt that was the thing Cromwell was depending on. He and Lambert had both seen a shortcoming in the adversary demeanors. They had focused such a large number of their soldiers on their traditional and therefore they were confined facing the coastline with little space to move whenever assaulted. The fact of the matter was, obviously, that they didn't anticipate being assaulted. They accepted that the drive was immovably in their grasp and this impression was affirmed during the evening of 2 September when they saw Cromwell draw up his powers in a cautious line behind the Broxburn, the little gorge what isolated the two militaries. After a couple of bogus alerts the two sides settled down for the evening — or so the Scots accepted. A large portion of the Scottish musketeers drenched their matches. In any case, all during that time of haziness Cromwell was working diligently putting together troop developments. One of his troopers saw him. 'Cromwell free all the night through the few regiments by torchlight, upon a little Scots bother, gnawing his lips till the blood ran down his jaw without his seeing it.' Fortunately it was a tempestuous, blustery evening and this assisted with hiding the secretive development from the ears of an arrogant opponent.

By sunrise six mounted force regiments and three and a half regiments of foot had crossed the precarious and dangerous slants of the Broxburn. It had been a troublesome and challenging move, however it worked impeccably. Their day break assault got the Scots not well ready. All things considered the adversary actually had a two to one benefit in numbers and there came a crucial time when the English line started to give ground. However, toward the beginning of today it was Cromwell's fight, being

battled on his conditions, and he was prepared with four regiments for possible later use. The effect of this sublimely coordinated second wave assault won the day. For one English official it was a remarkable second. 'The sun showing up upon the ocean I heard Noll say, "Presently let God emerge and his adversaries will be dispersed".' There was some furious battling at push of pike, however not for long. Inside an hour or so the Scots were in head-first retreat, 'driven', as one author put it, 'similar to turkeys by the English troopers'. As per Cromwell's own gauge 3000 Scots were killed and 10,000 taken prisoner; likewise caught were their cannons and stuff train. Like generally great commanders Cromwell took on the majority of his conflicts when he stood firm on the benefit of situation or numbers, or both. At Dunbar on 2 September 1650 all that appeared to be against him; yet by the following morning he had grabbed triumph from the grip of a skillful and experienced general. Who can fault the Scottish evangelist who said that Cromwell was more terrible than the Devil, 'For the sacred writing said, Resist the Devil and he will flie from you — however oppose Oliver and he will flie in your face.'

After Dunbar Leslie had too couple of men to hold Edinburgh so he pulled out to Stirling, the stronghold passage to the Highlands. Cromwell entered the Scottish capital on 7 September, however not until 24 December did the actual palace give up to a blend of gunnery discharge and discretion. Its authority, Dundas, soon a while later joined Cromwell's side, and this empowered the revolting Heath to see that the probably secure palace, until now known as the Maiden ought to from here on out be known as the Prostitute. Truth be told Heath was off base. The Maiden had been taken previously, by Alexander Leslie in 1639.

The remainder of the pre-winter and winter of 1650 Cromwell gave to broadening his command over south Scotland, utilizing Leith as his main stock base. He was restless to win the altruism of the neighborhood populace and his fighters upheld him by being, by the principles of a multitude of occupation, strikingly respectful. Their ordinary church participation acquired the hesitant esteem of many — and this regardless of the various manners by which Scottish Presbyterians and Cromwell's Independents flagged their endorsement of a decent lesson: the previous by moaning, the last option by murmuring. A portion of the fortifications sent throughout the colder time of year and spring were less all around focused than Cromwell's veterans, yet 'honored be the Lord, we are improving them day by day, finding a lot of consolation from the Lord therein'.

y haggling as frequently as conceivable with the Presbyterian chiefs Cromwell would have liked to wean them away from their union with Charles II. It was indeed

a collusion which neither one of the sides had found as they would prefer. He was not by and large actually a for them model lord, while he, as far as it matters for him, had been embarrassed by his total reliance upon them. Subsequently it was generally detailed that he had invited the insight about Dunbar. 'After this loss they all viewed the King as one they would genuinely need,' composed Clarendon. With sharp political knowledge Cromwell had anticipated this in a letter composed on the day after Dunbar. 'Without a doubt it's plausible that the Kirk has done their do. I accept their King will set up upon his own score now, wherein he will track down numerous companions.' The improvement in Charles' position was represented by his crowning celebration at Scone on 1 January 1651. Not that this would have stressed Cromwell much. He had close to nothing however hatred for Charles. 'Provide him with a shoulder of lamb and a prostitute, that is all he really focuses on.' Nonetheless Charles turned into a valuable point of convergence for public faithfulness, and with a multitude of occupation on their dirt it was just regular that numerous Scots should go to him.

Throughout the colder time of year of 1650-1 there was irregular skirmishing while the English soldiers remained alive on a little cheddar and simply a desire for horse-meat. As in Ireland, not really set in stone to make the colder time of year break as short as could be expected. On 4 February the military walked towards Falkirk, however the climate was 'so stormy with wind, hail, snow and downpour' that they had no real option except to turn around. On their return Cromwell took to his bed immediately — not by virtue of the Edinburgh lady who guaranteed that she kept him entertained 'and gloated all over of it, and that he used to give her twenty shillings a period' — but since he was sick. Not until early June was he completely recuperated. To a limited extent this was his own issue. Albeit on the day after Dunbar he kept in touch with his significant other, 'I guarantee you, I grow an elderly person, and feel sicknesses old enough grandly taking upon me', he was over-restless to return to work and, therefore, a few evident recuperations were trailed by backslides. Over and over it was supposed that he had kicked the bucket. He, at the end of the day, accepted that he had been at death's door.

Cromwell was partial to demanding that he was not basic. 'Your administration needs not me: I am a helpless animal, and have been a dry bone.' Nonetheless while he was sick in the spring of 1651 the Scottish lobby wavered and floated unconvincingly. In reasonableness to Cromwell's subordinates it ought to be brought up that overcoming the Lowlands was a certain something, entering the Highlands another, and that they were currently looked by the issue which had crushed numerous prior English militaries. Without even a trace of genuine battling, a few of the officials' spouses came north on a visit, among them Frances

Lambert who then, at that point, needed to compose back to London requesting fine yard. 'I don't have anything to wear about my neck, and I dare not go uncovered, inspired by a paranoid fear of giving offense to delicate saints.'

On 19 June Cromwell took the field again at the top of an enormous armed force, however for the following a month there still appeared to be no chance of carrying the Scots to fight or of getting through their protection lines. Not in any event, when Cromwell raged a braced house inside full perspective on their military would the Scots permit themselves to be drawn out. It was clear sufficient that the Achilles' impact point of the Scottish position was Fife. If by some stroke of good luck Fife could be involved then Stirling would be cut off from its cause of provisions and its safeguards would need to come out and battle or starve. However, an arrival on the bank of Fife would imply huge dangers; the soldiers would be defenseless against assault before they had the opportunity to refocus. In a later letter Cromwell summarized the disappointed state of mind of that month. 'We can genuinely say, we were gone the extent that we could in our advice and activity, and we said to each other, we realized not what to do.' Finally, nonetheless, God guided Cromwell to take a chance.

On 17 July, 1500 men under Colonel Overton crossed the Forth in boats and set up a bridgehead at North Ferry on a tight, effortlessly shielded promontory. After three days he was joined by Lambert bringing more than four regiments. The convoluted land and/or water capable activity was finished just under the wire; a Scottish power connected with them even as the last mounted force regiment was landing. At first on edge, Lambert headed toward the assault when every one of his soldiers were aground and, at Inverkeithing, at the neck of the promontory, he won a fine victory.

When Leslie heard the news his initially thought was to progress against Lambert with his primary armed force, yet when he saw Cromwell starting to move off in pursuit behind him, he understood that he may be trapped in the open between two militaries and chose rather to remain at Stirling. Cromwell then, at that point, walked to Queens ship and sent the heft of his soldiers across the Forth. By August his attack weapons were battering at the entryways of Perth. Here, on that very day, he heard the news for which he had been pausing. Charles II and the Scottish armed force were traveling south, to increase the illustrious expectation in England. With Cromwell and the pick of the Commonwealth troops now north of the Firth they could expect some early triumphs against sub-par resistance, a gathering momentum of help from all who went against conservative tax assessment and Independency in religion, and afterward one major fight to win two realms at a stroke. It was a bet, obviously, however when Cromwell held Fife and Perth

their main choices were to stay at Stirling and be famished into accommodation, or to pull out into the Highlands and into political haziness. For Charles it was a bet definitely worth taking; as he told his devotees he 'had however a day to day existence to lose'. A letter composed by the Duke of Hamilton mirrors the disposition in the Royalist camp. 'We have stopped Scotland being hardly ready to keep up with it, but we handle by any means, and only all will fulfill us, or to lose all. I admit I can't let you know whether our expectations or fears are most prominent, however we have one heavy contention, despair; for we should either forcefully battle it, or bite the dust.' As it ended up, Hamilton was to do both.

Cromwell, paradoxically, was calmly certain. He got the acquiescence of Perth on 2 August and afterward got back to Leith. There he permitted his officers to rest for 48 hours and sent a consoling dispatch to Parliament wherein he transparently clarified the system of the campaign.

I do catch that if he [Charles] goes for England, being exactly couple of days walk before us, it will inconvenience a few men's musings, and may event a few burdens; of which I trust we are just about as profoundly reasonable as any; and for sure this is our solace, that in effortlessness of heart as to God, we have done to the best of our decisions, realizing that assuming some issue were not put to this business, it would event one more winter's conflict to the destruction of your soldiery, for whom the Scots are too hard in regard of bearing the colder time of year troubles of this nation, and been under the unending cost of the financier of England in indicting this conflict. It could be assumed we may have kept the adversary from this, by mediating among him and England; which really I accept we may: however how to eliminate him out of this spot, without doing what we have done, except if we had a telling armed force on the two sides of the waterway of Forth, isn't get to us.

Cromwell then, at that point, reminded his perusers free from the Battles of Preston, when 'upon intentional counsel, we picked rather to put ourselves between their military and Scotland: and how God succeeded that, isn't well to be neglected'. This time besides the Scots were attacking with a more modest armed force and had taken their choice, as Cromwell wrote 'in distress and dread, and out of inescapable need'. The Scots were attacking, however Cromwell held the drive. He had opened a brilliant scaffold for them, and they had crossed it, realizing that they were walking into a snare, and knowing likewise that there was nothing else they could do. Also all things considered, had not simply the incomparable Cromwell been caught at Dunbar?

But, in contrast to the Scots at Dunbar, Cromwell was in no rush to come down

off the slope. He left Monck (presently a Lieutenant-General) with 6000 men and orders to take Stirling. He sent Lambert ahead with the rangers to shadow and bug the Scots, while different powers under Harrison, Fleetwood, Desborough and Fairfax — presently untroubled by second thoughts — were accumulated in status in England. Then, at that point, on 6 August Cromwell left Leith. At that point Charles had effectively crossed the Border. The following not many weeks were sharply frustrating for the youthful King. In spite of the fact that he walked through customarily Royalist regions, Lancashire and the Welsh Marches, the normal help didn't come in. Recalling the looting of 1648 even dedicated Royalists were hesitant to help what looked dubiously like a Scottish attack. On 22 August, blue and depleted, the King's military — perhaps 16,000 strong — stopped at Worcester.

y that date Cromwell's infantry, walking south on an equal course, had as of now arrived at Nottingham. Not until his arrangements were finished had Cromwell left Scotland, however at that point he moved quick. His troopers were permitted to walk in their shirtsleeves, their external dress and weapons being continued horseback. When he arrived at Evesham, on 27 August, Cromwell could rely on in excess of 30,000 troopers. With such overpowering prevalence in numbers he could bear over partition his military. Fleetwood and Lambert toward the south and west of Worcester hindered all chance of retreat into Wales; Cromwell toward the east stood with on leg on each side of the way to London. Worcester was encircled. Cromwell moved in for the final blow. He put his gunnery on Red Hill and on 29 August they started shooting. For the following four days Cromwell paused. To complete his arrangement of assault he expected to gather an adequate number of boats to fabricate two extensions; yet conceivably he was likewise hanging tight for something different: 3 September, the commemoration of Dunbar. As he rode around assessing his officers he 'was engaged with a bounty of euphoria by unprecedented yelling from each regiment, troop and friends as he went to show respect to them'.

On the morning of 3 September everything was prepared. The field-word that day was 'the Lord of Hosts' — as it had been at Dunbar. Fleetwood's errand was to put the two scaffolds in position, inside a gun fired of one another, one over the Severn, the other across the Teme. This would permit his and Cromwell's armed forces to join and progress on Worcester from the west, drawing the net even more firmly. To forestall this combination of powers the Royalists emerged from the city, yet were moved back by sheer weight of numbers. Then, at that point, as Cromwell composed, 'we beat the foe from one fence to another till we beat him into Worcester'. Presently totally trimmed in, Charles drove a last desperate

sally against the eastern piece of Cromwell's military, still on Red Hill. It almost worked, however Lambert and Harrison hung on long enough to give time for Cromwell to get back over the Severn by the scaffold of boats. This settled the matter. The Royalists contended energetically. 'For four or five hours,' composed Cromwell, 'it was as firm a challenge as ever I have seen.' When ammo ran out, the Royalist musketeers utilized their firearms as clubs. However, squeezed from two bearings on the double they were crashed once more into Worcester and tracked down their own cannons, expected to guard the city, betrayed them.

Bitter and confounded road battling proceeded until into the evening. Nearly 2000 of Charles' fighters were killed there. 'What with the dead assemblages of men and the dead ponies of the foe filling the roads, there was such a terribleness that a man could scarcely stand the town,' composed Major-General Harrison. Charles and 4000 others got away and escaped; the rest were taken prisoner. In a progression of experiences including camouflage, ministers' openings and the legal oak tree, Charles advanced toward Brighton and afterward to France. In transit he let a metalworker know who was shoeing his pony that the difficulty was all the shortcoming of that rebel Charles Stuart for acquiring the Scots. He didn't commit that error next time.

Worcester denoted the peak of Cromwell's tactical vocation. He, when all is said and done, portrayed it as 'a delegated kindness'. He never again took the field at the top of his military. His ten swarmed years were finished. Barely any officers rose so quick or accomplished such a great amount in so short a time.

9. This Extraordinary Man

As a compensation for his works Parliament gave Cromwell Hampton Court as a home — and it turned into an end of the week house where he and his family could get away from the considerations of state. Albeit in principle the Rump was sovereign, progressively men had come to look to Cromwell. 'Incredible things' thought of one solicitor, 'God has done by you in war, and beneficial things men anticipate from you in harmony: to break in pieces the oppressor, to facilitate the mistreated of their weights, to deliver the detainees out of bonds, and to alleviate helpless families with bread.' As their terrified response to the bits of gossip about Cromwell's demise in Scotland shows, even the individuals from the Rump knew where the truth of force lay. There was an error between the sacred form

— he House of Commons — and the truth of force — Cromwell's military. However bringing structure and reality into closer understanding was offensive to the individuals from the Rump. It would mean the finish of what impact they had: in addition a significant number of them were persuaded Republicans and regretted anything which resembled placing the public authority under the control of a solitary individual, regardless of whether King or Commander-in-Chief. Then again, how should the Rump perhaps guarantee to address individuals? They were in the Commons on the grounds that their names had not been on Colonel Pride's rundown, and the House of Commons was there in light of the fact that it had not been canceled when the government and the House of Lords were nullified in 1649. At the point when England turned into a Republic no new constitution had been set up;

men essentially managed with the fag-end of the former one.It was an exceptionally unsuitable situation and, accordingly, barely anything was finished. The military turned out to be increasingly eager. Cromwell trusted that the Rump of the Long Parliament would break down itself and grant new decisions on a more evenhanded establishment. However, as time elapsed it turned out to be progressively evident that the Rump could never go willingly. 'Do you mean to stay here till Armageddon come?' went a number of the time. The arrangement was self-evident, however as Cromwell said, the possibility of it made his 'hair remain on end'. In the long run, in April 1653 when the Rump appeared to be very nearly passing an Act to delay its reality even further, his understanding snapped. He went to the House and paid attention to the discussion for some time. Then, at that point, he leant across to Major-General Harrison. 'This is the time I should do it,' he murmured. Removing his cap, he rose and started to talk, at first smoothly and reasonably. Yet, soon his annoyance and disappointment burst through. He blamed the

individuals for bad form and personal responsibility, of corruptly sticking on to office. As his attitude rose he started to single out people, pointing at them as he yelled out their issues; this one a reprobate, that an alcoholic, a third bad. He strolled about as he talked, set his cap back on, kicked the ground irately. Then, at that point, at the stature of what seemed, by all accounts, to be a wild angry outburst, he conveyed his sentence on them. 'Maybe you imagine that this isn't parliamentary language: I admit it isn't; nor are you to anticipate any from me. You are no parliament, I say you are no parliament. I will stop your sitting. Call them in.' Here he went to Harrison who left the Chamber and reemerged with twenty or thirty musketeers. As the individuals were hustled out Cromwell checked out the mace lying on the table before the Speaker. 'How will we manage this doodad? Here remove it.' And in this way, after his very own design, Cromwell broke up Parliament.

Now the Commons had been abrogated as well. The main appropriately established expert in the realm was Cromwell, as Commander-in-Chief. To his foes it in some cases appeared to be that Cromwell had arranged this from the start. 'In the entirety of his progressions he planned only to propel himself.' truth be told he had followed up spontaneously and observed his new position humiliating. His first response was to hand his power over to another person — to a designated gathering of 140 men which came to be known as Barebones' Parliament, after one of the individuals for London, a calfskin vender and Baptist

— raisegod Barebones by name. Be that as it may, this gathering contained a gathering of extremists which was sufficiently huge to make a great deal of clamor and once in a while to compromise personal stakes, for example, the lawful calling and the nation noble man's control of area issues. By December 1653 the more safe individuals were so frightened by different extremist proposition that they chose to disintegrate themselves and hand their position back to Cromwell … Some of the revolutionaries attempted to carry on like nothing had occurred except for by and by officers were shipped off the House. When asked by the Colonel responsible for the activity what they were doing there, they answered 'We are looking for the Lord'. 'Then, at that point,' he said, 'you might go somewhere else, for to my specific information he has not been here these last twelve years.'After this Cromwell looked up to the way that he was the main man in the country who could order the help of both the military and the nation nobility. In December 1653 he accepted the title of Lord Protector. 'As such,' composed Clarendon, 'and with so little agonies, this phenomenal man against the longings of generally respectable people or men of value mounted himself

upon the high position of three realms, without the name of lord however with a more noteworthy power and authority than ever practiced or asserted by any ruler.' At him he had a military and naval force far bigger than the powers accessible to any past English ruler. They were paid for by tax collection at a level higher than that which had assisted with causing the resistance in any case. Despite the fact that the need to keep up with multitudes of occupation in Ireland and Scotland secured no less than 25,000 troopers, the impression of extraordinary strength

— ver all maritime strength — was adequate to make conceivable a wide-running and forceful unfamiliar policy.

hen Cromwell became Lord Protector he assumed control over an administration at battle with the Dutch. It was a conflict directed exclusively by trade interests and he objected to it. In April 1654 he wiped the slate clean. It wasn't so much that that he was apathetic regarding the necessities of England's sea trade. Exchange wars sounded good to him, however he felt that it should be feasible to join exchange and religion a conflict against the heathens or Catholics. Right off the bat in 1654 he sent Admiral Blake to the Mediterranean. His errand was to offer the weapons of his armada as a powerful influence for any individual who had been causing problems for English traders. As regular Blake did all that was requested from him. It was the start of British gunboat strategy in the Mediterranean.

In the mid year of 1654 Cromwell turned with excitement to a task expected to break the Spanish imposing business model in the West Indies and Central America. Cromwell called it 'broadening the limits of Christ's realm'. Tragically Cromwell's consultants persuaded him to think that it would be a simple undertaking and subsequently the campaign was gravely bungled beginning to end. The assault on Hispaniola fizzled, and albeit a little province was set up in Jamaica it floated for a long time near the precarious edge of breakdown. Different plans to force individuals to become homesteaders failed to work out. The London massage parlors were assaulted and 400 whores gathered together yet they were not all things considered, as had been by and large anticipated, shipped off Jamaica. Furthermore it was remarkably difficult to track down anybody to go willingly to a district where illness and war took such a substantial toll.

Undoubtedly Cromwell should assume some liability for the deficient arrangements, and he knew it. At the point when he knew about the disaster in Hispaniola, he shut himself up in his space for an entire day, agonizing over the catastrophe. However the settlement on Jamaica made due to turn into a focal point of the slave exchange and a turn of British supreme and international strategy in the eighteenth century. The far off results of this most incompetent scene were pivotal. As of now in

Cromwell's the very beginning pamphleteer made plain that behind the discussion of a Protestant mission there were different interests working. 'Our shippers they travel via ocean and land to make Christian converts, yet think about their practices, and the benefit we have by their misleading, first in denying the helpless Indians of that which God hath given them, and afterward bringing of it home to us.'

because of the assault on the West Indies Cromwell ended up associated with an European conflict with Spain. For Cromwell war implied attacking. In March 1657 he consented to help the French in an assault on the Spanish Netherlands, an assault which would strike at the base from which Charles II expected to dispatch another attack. Cromwell was to supply a multitude of 6000 men and his award was to be the cession of Mardyck and Dunkirk (when caught). This ought to have implied more powerful control of the Channel and 'an entryway into the landmass'. After his West Indies experience Cromwell went to considerable lengths to oversee the arrangements more closely.

In May the expeditionary power arrived at Boulogne and was put under the general order of the incomparable French Marshal Turenne. In the missions of 1657 and 1658 the contrasts between the mainland and English styles of fighting turned out to be extremely evident. 'Battling isn't a lot of the design in these parts,' thought of one English authority who had a satiate of drawn-out attack operations.

At the attack of Ypres Major-General Morgan recommended to Turenne that they should storm the outworks of this very much braced city. Turenne, the expert specialist, was horrified.

He] gazed upward towards the sky and said 'Did ever my lord, the King of

France, or the King of Spain, endeavor a counterscarp upon an attack where there were three half-moons covered with gun, and the defenses of the town playing point clear into the counterscarp? What will the King my lord consider me, on the off chance that I open his military to these risks?' And he ascended, and fell into an enthusiasm, stepping with his feet, and shaking his locks and smiling with his teeth, he said Major-General Morgan had made him mad.

But in the long run Morgan was allowed to attempt and, obviously, the counterscarp was taken and Ypres gave up when its own weapons were betrayed it. In the main pitched clash of the missions, the Battle of the Dunes (right external Dunkirk) in June 1658, the English infantry again separated themselves. To assault the Spanish position they needed to scramble up a sandhill on all fours. Be that as it may, they did it. At the top the

musketeers terminated two volleys and afterward the winded pikemen evened out their pikes and charged home. This was the unequivocal second in the fight. After ten days Dunkirk gave up. Not long before the two militaries conflicted, Turenne and his staff had been alarmed to hear an extraordinary yell from the English detachment; they rode over to get some information about. Morgan replied, 'It was the typical custom of the Red-coats, when they saw the foe, to celebrate.' Turenne was by all account not the only one to be dazzled. Cromwell's military and naval force implied that Cromwell had become, as the Duke of Tuscany put it, 'the fear of the entire world'. Indeed, even the Royalist Clarendon conceded that 'Cromwell's significance at home was a simple shadow of his significance abroad'. In Dryden's expression, he had encouraged the British Lion to thunder. It was a long ways from the situation in 1640 when, as the Venetian minister composed, England had turned into 'a country futile to the remainder of the world, and thusly of no consideration'.

Three months after his military's triumph at the Battle of the Dunes Cromwell passed on at Whitehall on 3 September 1658, the commemoration of Dunbar and Worcester. 'It satisfied the Lord, on this day to take him to rest, it having in the past been a day of works to him.'

His work didn't long endure him. His picked replacement, his child Richard, had none of the characteristics which were expected to hold together an arrangement of government unsanctified by custom. With the death of the man whose individual characteristics alone had made it work, the delicate Cromwellian framework separated and cleared a path for the arrival of conventional specialists and customary qualities. To praise this Restoration

Cromwell's body was uncovered. For a really long time it hung from the scaffold of Tyburn, then, at that point, the cadaver was brought down and beheaded.

Even when dead Cromwell excited overwhelming inclinations and right up 'til today he has stayed at the focal point of discussion. It isn't important to be an antiquarian to pass judgment on oneself to be either Roundhead or Cavalier by demeanor and, subsequently, to arrange either possibly in support of Cromwell. Also for Roundheads like the writer of this book, there is an extra issue. They realize that they would have ridden next to Cromwell at Naseby and would have partaken in his temperament of inebriated thrill on that day, however on whose side would they have been at Burford when he squashed the Levelers in the military? Moderate, liberal, revolutionary, fundamentalist — this large number of names and more have been attached to Cromwell the legislator. However, about Cromwell the officer there can be no question. To pick a World XI of Great Generals and contend about

Cromwell's position in the batting request would be a purposeless exercise; the reality stays that he was an extraordinary leader. It isn't only that he won fights and conveyed each mission to an effective end. Throughout his vocation he displayed in England that he could deal with rangers in the hotness of fight preferred considerably over Prince Rupert; he displayed in Ireland that he was an expert of attack fighting with a decent eye for the employments of ocean power; he showed, in Scotland, that in any event, when dwarfed and in a substandard position he could summon triumph out of up and coming loss. When, at the Council of War at Hodder Bridge in August 1648, he took his first significant key choice, he showed that he was not terrified of the reasonable courses of action. In his quest for the Scots after Preston he showed a persistent assurance to commute home each benefit. Assuming that absolute triumph were conceivable then triumph alone was adequately not. Definitiveness in looking for the fight to come and a controlled savagery in pursuit — these were to be his trademarks as a general.

But Cromwell was something other than a fine warrior. His exceptional quality was that he saw more unmistakably than any of his peers the chance of pursuing another sort of battle in a nation where the strongholds were a few hundred years obsolete. He saw that the standards of seventeenth-century fighting, rules fitting to mainland conditions, were, in England, rules which could be broken. Consequently not until the foe powers in the field had been squashed did he fret about the catch of towns. It is possible that he was helped by going to the conflict liberated from those biases which definitely existed in the personalities of more experienced officials — the previously established inclinations dependent on crusades abroad. As a regular citizen in 1642 he would have shared the overall view that the conflict would be a short one, though a portion of the expert officers who came to England right now accepted that it could well keep going for a long time. Then, at that point, as time elapsed, as tax assessment expanded and the social request started to separate, Cromwell the legislator more likely than not become all the more definitely mindful of the requirement for another sort of fighting. As the expectation of a short conflict blurred, so the requirement for it developed more pressing. This to be sure was the message which Cromwell explained in his discourse of 9 December 1644, the renowned discourse on the Self-Denying Ordinance.

It is currently an opportunity to talk, or always hold the tongue. The significant event presently is no not exactly to save a Nation out of a dying, nay, practically kicking the bucket condition, which the long continuation of this War hath currently brought it into; so that without a more expedient, vivacious and efficacious indictment of the War — pushing off all waiting procedures like those of

officers of-fortune past ocean, to turn out a conflict — we will make the Kingdom exhausted of us, and disdain the name of Parliament.

As a legislator who needed to legitimize the undeniable degree of war tax assessment, who assisted with doing a regulatory transformation in the Eastern Association, Cromwell felt more forcefully than did most fighters the tensions which requested a rapid finish to everything. Subsequently albeit some tactical antiquarians, quite those history specialists who are themselves officers, see him with aversion as an in warrior issues of state, as a trooper with the shrewd psyche of a government official, touchy to shifts in the nation's mind-set — in this so in contrast to their courageous saint, Sir Thomas Fairfax — it might well have been definitively this 'unsoldierly' side to his person which made him so momentous a soldier.

ut the forceful, Napoleonic style of fighting which he took on set extraordinary expectations for the confidence and discipline of his soldiers. At Dunbar following six dampening a long time of an evidently unbeneficial crusade in troubling climate, they were relied upon to dispatch a night assault on a mathematically prevalent and very much posted foe. However they did it. At Preston, after a long walk from south west Wales and a hard fight, they were relied upon to continue to battle for two additional days until the Scots were crashed into the ground. Furthermore they did it. At Langport his cavalry was relied upon to make an evidently self-destructive charge uphill along a tight path. They did it and its shock won the fight. Consistently Cromwell's cavalry opposed the impulse to dissipate in quest for an escaping foe. With men like this Cromwell could bear to face challenges which in different officers would have been frenzy. He had motivation to be glad for his 'wonderful organization'. What's more undeniably it was his organization. In contrast to a portion of his more highborn counterparts, he didn't accept central leadership right toward the start of his profession. He began as skipper of a troop and from that point he moved gradually up, totally on his benefits. The years 1642-4 saw not just his own tactical apprenticeship, they saw likewise the fashioning of the instrument with which the Civil War was won: the rangers regiments of the Eastern Association and the New Model Army. This also was to a great extent Cromwell's work. In January 1645 a regiment undermined rebellion on hearing that it was to be put under another officer. In this connection among him and his men he had a benefit denied to, for instance, a generally skilful general like Waller. Along these lines, independently in 1642-4, he made himself remarkably all around set to battle the sort of war which was fitting to English conditions. The arrangements of the Self-Denying Ordinance could

not reasonably be concerned with him. As Sir Thomas Fairfax acknowledged, Cromwell could deal with a military well since he had assisted with making it.

hanks generally to this twofold accomplishment Parliament won the Civil Wars — a result which was in no way, shape or form an inevitable outcome. Then, at that point, as Lord Protector, Cromwell pushed open the entryway prompting England's future as a maritime power. The artist Edmund Waller, in lines committed to Cromwell, proposes a developing public pride.

The ocean's our own; and presently all
countries welcome With twisting sails every
vessel of our armada; Your power stretches
out the extent that breezes can blow Or
enlarging sails upon the globe may go.

Soldier, legislator, legislator — hence the men with whom he is most much of the time thought about are Caesar and Napoleon, however in numerous ways there is a nearer equal in the vocation of the incomparable Czech general, John Zizka. Every one of them in the final hotel owed their ascent to their tactical ability. For Cromwell's situation, given the conditions of the initial forty years of his life, this was a remarkable, practically mystifying ability. In any case, similar to it or not — and more likely than not the suspected would have been hostile to him — this devout, sloppy, moderately aged country man of honor came to live by the blade. Hence it is not really shocking that he ought to be most distinctively recalled in Ireland, where his blade's edge was at its most honed. To see him through Irish eyes, nonetheless, is to see him in a mirror twisted by the occasions of ensuing hundreds of years, and assuming we surrender to the wizardry of that fantasy we neglect to see the diserse significance of the man — a man who, when he needed to, could dispose of conventional things, similar to lords and rules of war.

Acknowledgments

Ashmolean Museum, Oxford British Museum, London Bibliothèque National, Paris Cromwell Museum, Huntingdon Gemeentemusea van Deventer Kimbolton School, Huntingdonshire National Army Museum, London National Portrait Gallery, London Radio Times Hulton Picture Library Society of Antiquaries of London Weidenfeld and Nicolson Archives

Select Bibliography

The best history is C. H. Firth, Oliver Cromwell and the Rule of the Puritans in England (1900). Likewise great are C. Slope, God's Englishman: Oliver Cromwell and the English Revolution (1970) and A. Fraser, Cromwell Our Chief of Men (1973).

C. H. Firth, Cromwell's Army (1902) is deservedly the standard work regarding this matter, however for the extremely significant re-association of the powers of the Eastern Association it should be enhanced by C. Holmes, The Eastern Association in the English Civil War (1974). On the Royalist Army see: I. Roy, The Royalist Army in the First Civil War (forthcoming).

S. R. Gardiner, History of the Great Civil War, 4 vols (1886-91) is a fine definite story. Comprehensible reviews are C.V. Wedgwood, The King's War

1641-1647 (1958), P. Youthful and R. Holmes, The English Civil War (1974),
. Woolrych, Battles of the English Civil War (1966) and A. H. Burne and P.
Youthful, The Great Civil War (1959).

On Cromwell himself there are the old investigations by T.S. Baldock, Cromwell as a Soldier (1899) and W. S. Douglas, Cromwell's Scotch Campaigns (1899). Other common conflict commanders have been better off, for instance, F.T.R. Edgar, Sir Ralph Hopton (1968), J. Adair, Roundhead General. A tactical account of Sir William Waller (1969) and M. Ashley, Cromwell's Generals (1954).

The most valuable book on seventeenth-century fighting on the landmass is G. Parker, The Army of Flanders and the Spanish Road (1972). An animating hypothesis is propounded by M. Roberts in The Military Revolution 1560-1660 (1955).

n common conflict fortresses in England see: Royal Commission on Historical Monuments: Newark on Trent (1964).

A beginning has been made on the fundamental work of setting the Civil War in the more extensive system of English society: I. Roy, 'The English Civil War and English Society' in War and Society. A Yearbook of Military History. Vol. I (1975).